This report contains the collective views of international groups of experts and does not necessarily represent the decisions or the stated policy of the United Nations Environment Programme, the International Labour Organization, or the World Health Organization.

Environmental Health Criteria 228

PRINCIPLES AND METHODS FOR THE ASSESSMENT OF RISK FROM ESSENTIAL TRACE ELEMENTS

Published under the joint sponsorship of the United Nations Environment Programme, the International Labour Organization, and the World Health Organization, and produced within the framework of the Inter-Organization Programme for the Sound Management of Chemicals.

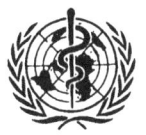

World Health Organization
Geneva, 2002

The **International Programme on Chemical Safety (IPCS)**, established in 1980, is a joint venture of the United Nations Environment Programme (UNEP), the International Labour Organization (ILO), and the World Health Organization (WHO). The overall objectives of the IPCS are to establish the scientific basis for assessment of the risk to human health and the environment from exposure to chemicals, through international peer-review processes, as a prerequisite for the promotion of chemical safety, and to provide technical assistance in strengthening national capacities for the sound management of chemicals.

The **Inter-Organization Programme for the Sound Management of Chemicals (IOMC)** was established in 1995 by UNEP, ILO, the Food and Agriculture Organization of the United Nations, WHO, the United Nations Industrial Development Organization, the United Nations Institute for Training and Research, and the Organisation for Economic Co-operation and Development (Participating Organizations), following recommendations made by the 1992 UN Conference on Environment and Development to strengthen cooperation and increase coordination in the field of chemical safety. The purpose of the IOMC is to promote coordination of the policies and activities pursued by the Participating Organizations, jointly or separately, to achieve the sound management of chemicals in relation to human health and the environment.

WHO Library Cataloguing-in-Publication Data

Principles and methods for the assessment of risk from essential trace elements.

(Environmental health criteria ; 228)

1.Trace elements – adverse effects 2.Nutritional requirements 3.Homeostasis
4.Maximum allowable concentration 5.Risk assessment
I.International Programme on Chemical Safety II.Series

ISBN 92 4 157228 0   (NLM Classification: QU 130)
ISSN 0250-863X

The World Health Organization welcomes requests for permission to reproduce or translate its publications, in part or in full. Applications and enquiries should be addressed to the Office of Publications, World Health Organization, Geneva, Switzerland, which will be glad to provide the latest information on any changes made to the text, plans for new editions, and reprints and translations already available.

©World Health Organization 2001

Publications of the World Health Organization enjoy copyright protection in accordance with the provisions of Protocol 2 of the Universal Copyright Convention. All rights reserved.

The designations employed and the presentation of the material in this publication do not imply the expression of any opinion whatsoever on the part of the Secretariat of the World Health Organization concerning the legal status of any country, territory, city or area or of its authorities, or concerning the delimitation of its frontiers or boundaries.

The mention of specific companies or of certain manufacturers' products does not imply that they are endorsed or recommended by the World Health Organization in preference to others of a similar nature that are not mentioned. Errors and omissions excepted, the names of proprietary products are distinguished by initial capital letters.

The Federal Ministry for the Environment, Nature Conservation and Nuclear Safety, Germany, provided financial support for, and undertook the printing of, this publication.

Computer typesetting by I. Xavier Lourduraj, Chennai, India

CONTENTS

ENVIRONMENTAL HEALTH CRITERIA FOR
PRINCIPLES AND METHODS FOR THE ASSESSMENT
OF RISK FROM ESSENTIAL TRACE ELEMENTS

1. SUMMARY 1

2. INTRODUCTION 3

    2.1 Scope and purpose 3
    2.2 Criteria for essentiality of trace elements 5
        2.2.1 Essentiality and homeostatic mechanisms .. 6
    2.3 Terminology 6
        2.3.1 Definitions relating to individual and
              population requirements for ETEs 7
            2.3.1.1 Factorial estimation of nutrient
                    requirement 7
            2.3.1.2 Requirements for the individual ... 7
            2.3.1.3 Dietary reference intakes, popu-
                    lation reference intakes, reference
                    nutrient intakes, recommended
                    dietary allowance, and safe range
                    of population mean intake 8
        2.3.2 Toxicological terms 10
            2.3.2.1 Acceptable daily intake, toler-
                    able intake, tolerable upper intake
                    level 10
            2.3.2.2 Reference dose 10
        2.3.3 Principles underlying derivation of nutri-
              ent requirements and tolerable intakes 10
        2.3.4 Approaches to define a threshold dose ... 11
        2.3.5 Characteristics of uncertainty factors 12
        2.3.6 Estimating TI from dose–response
              curve for critical effect 14

3. THE ACCEPTABLE RANGE OF ORAL INTAKE
   FOR AN ESSENTIAL TRACE ELEMENT 16

    3.1 Definition of an AROI 16

	3.2	Boundaries of an AROI 17
		3.2.1 Lower limit of an AROI 18
		3.2.2 Upper limit of an AROI 18
	3.3	Comparison of safety evaluations 20

4. VARIABILITY OF HUMAN POPULATIONS 22

    4.1 Principles of homeostasis of ETEs in humans 22
    4.2 Bioavailability 24
         4.2.1 Bioavailability and utilization 25
    4.3 Age-related variables 25
         4.3.1 *In utero* 25
         4.3.2 Infancy 27
         4.3.3 The elderly 27
    4.4 Variability due to gender 28
    4.5 Pregnancy and lactation 28
    4.6 Chemical species of ETEs 29
    4.7 Interactions between ETEs 30
         4.7.1 Copper and zinc 30
         4.7.2 Selenium and iodine 31
    4.8 Genetically determined human variability and
         disorders of homeostasis 31
    4.9 Acquired disorders of homeostasis 32

5. EFFECTS OF DEFICIENCY AND EXCESS 33

    5.1 Range in severity of effects 33
    5.2 Comparability of end-points used to define
         deficiency and excess 33
         5.2.1 Range of clinical and biochemical
                markers of deficiency and excess 35
                5.2.1.1 Deficiency 35
                5.2.1.2 Excess 35
         5.2.2 Examples of range of effects 36
                5.2.2.1 Iron 36
                5.2.2.2 Zinc 37
                5.2.2.3 Copper 38
                5.2.2.4 Selenium 38

6. APPLICATION OF HOMEOSTATIC MODEL IN HUMAN HEALTH RISK ASSESSMENT TO EXPOSURE TO ETEs 40

    6.1   Summary of principles 40
    6.2   Scheme for application of principles 42

7. RECOMMENDATIONS 46

8. FURTHER RESEARCH 47

REFERENCES 48

RESUME 57

RESUMEN 59

NOTE TO READERS OF THE CRITERIA MONOGRAPHS

Every effort has been made to present information in the criteria monographs as accurately as possible without unduly delaying their publication. In the interest of all users of the Environmental Health Criteria monographs, readers are requested to communicate any errors that may have occurred to the Director of the International Programme on Chemical Safety, World Health Organization, Geneva, Switzerland, in order that they may be included in corrigenda.

* * *

A detailed data profile and a legal file can be obtained from the International Register of Potentially Toxic Chemicals, Case postale 356, 1219 Châtelaine, Geneva, Switzerland (telephone no. + 41 22 - 9799111, fax no. + 41 22 - 7973460, E-mail irptc@unep.ch).

* * *

This publication was made possible by grant number 5 U01 ES02617-15 from the National Institute of Environmental Health Sciences, National Institutes of Health, USA, and by financial support from the Ministry of Health, Chile, and the European Commission.

Environmental Health Criteria

PREAMBLE

Objectives

In 1973 the WHO Environmental Health Criteria Programme was initiated with the following objectives:

(i) to assess information on the relationship between exposure to environmental pollutants and human health, and to provide guidelines for setting exposure limits;

(ii) to identify new or potential pollutants;

(iii) to identify gaps in knowledge concerning the health effects of pollutants;

(iv) to promote the harmonization of toxicological and epidemiological methods in order to have internationally comparable results.

The first Environmental Health Criteria (EHC) monograph, on mercury, was published in 1976 and since that time an ever-increasing number of assessments of chemicals and of physical effects have been produced. In addition, many EHC monographs have been devoted to evaluating toxicological methodology, e.g. for genetic, neurotoxic, teratogenic and nephrotoxic effects. Other publications have been concerned with epidemiological guidelines, evaluation of short-term tests for carcinogens, biomarkers, effects on the elderly and so forth.

Since its inauguration the EHC Programme has widened its scope, and the importance of environmental effects, in addition to health effects, has been increasingly emphasized in the total evaluation of chemicals.

The original impetus for the Programme came from World Health Assembly resolutions and the recommendations of the 1972 UN Conference on the Human Environment. Subsequently the work became an integral part of the International Programme on Chemical Safety (IPCS), a cooperative programme of UNEP, ILO and WHO. In this manner, with the strong support of the new partners, the importance of occupational health and environmental effects was fully recognized. The EHC monographs have become widely established, used and recognized throughout the world.

The recommendations of the 1992 UN Conference on Environment and Development and the subsequent establishment of the Intergovernmental Forum on Chemical Safety with the priorities for action in the six programme areas of Chapter 19, Agenda 21, all lend further weight to the need for EHC assessments of the risks of chemicals.

Scope

The criteria monographs are intended to provide critical reviews on the effect on human health and the environment of chemicals and of combinations of chemicals and physical and biological agents. As such, they include and review studies that are of direct relevance for the evaluation. However, they do not describe *every* study carried out. Worldwide data are used and are quoted from original studies, not from abstracts or reviews. Both published and unpublished reports are considered and it is incumbent on the authors to assess all the articles cited in the references. Preference is always given to published data. Unpublished data are used only when relevant published data are absent or when they are pivotal to the risk assessment. A detailed policy statement is available that describes the procedures used for unpublished proprietary data so that this information can be used in the evaluation without compromising its confidential nature (WHO (1999) Guidelines for the Preparation of Environmental Health Criteria. PCS/99.9, Geneva, World Health Organization).

In the evaluation of human health risks, sound human data, whenever available, are preferred to animal data. Animal and *in vitro* studies provide support and are used mainly to supply evidence missing from human studies. It is mandatory that research on human subjects is conducted in full accord with ethical principles, including the provisions of the Helsinki Declaration.

The EHC monographs are intended to assist national and international authorities in making risk assessments and subsequent risk management decisions. They represent a thorough evaluation of risks and are not, in any sense, recommendations for regulation or standard setting. These latter are the exclusive purview of national and regional governments.

Content

The layout of EHC monographs for chemicals is outlined below.

- Summary – a review of the salient facts and the risk evaluation of the chemical
- Identity – physical and chemical properties, analytical methods
- Sources of exposure
- Environmental transport, distribution and transformation
- Environmental levels and human exposure
- Kinetics and metabolism in laboratory animals and humans
- Effects on laboratory mammals and *in vitro* test systems
- Effects on humans
- Effects on other organisms in the laboratory and field
- Evaluation of human health risks and effects on the environment
- Conclusions and recommendations for protection of human health and the environment
- Further research
- Previous evaluations by international bodies, e.g. IARC, JECFA, JMPR

Selection of chemicals

Since the inception of the EHC Programme, the IPCS has organized meetings of scientists to establish lists of priority chemicals for subsequent evaluation. Such meetings have been held in Ispra, Italy, 1980; Oxford, United Kingdom, 1984; Berlin, Germany, 1987; and North Carolina, USA, 1995. The selection of chemicals has been based on the following criteria: the existence of scientific evidence that the substance presents a hazard to human health and/or the environment; the possible use, persistence, accumulation or degradation of the substance shows that there may be significant human or environmental exposure; the size and nature of populations at risk (both human and other species) and risks for environment; international concern, i.e. the substance is of major interest to several countries; adequate data on the hazards are available.

If an EHC monograph is proposed for a chemical not on the priority list, the IPCS Secretariat consults with the Cooperating Organizations and all the Participating Institutions before embarking on the preparation of the monograph.

Procedures

The order of procedures that result in the publication of an EHC monograph is shown in the flow chart on p. xi. A designated staff member of IPCS, responsible for the scientific quality of the document, serves as Responsible Officer (RO). The IPCS Editor is responsible for layout and language. The first draft, prepared by consultants or, more usually, staff from an IPCS Participating Institution, is based initially on data provided from the International Register of Potentially Toxic Chemicals, and reference data bases such as Medline and Toxline.

The draft document, when received by the RO, may require an initial review by a small panel of experts to determine its scientific quality and objectivity. Once the RO finds the document acceptable as a first draft, it is distributed, in its unedited form, to well over 150 EHC contact points throughout the world who are asked to comment on its completeness and accuracy and, where necessary, provide additional material. The contact points, usually designated by governments, may be Participating Institutions, IPCS Focal Points, or individual scientists known for their particular expertise. Generally some four months are allowed before the comments are considered by the RO and author(s). A second draft incorporating comments received and approved by the Director, IPCS, is then distributed to Task Group members, who carry out the peer review, at least six weeks before their meeting.

The Task Group members serve as individual scientists, not as representatives of any organization, government or industry. Their function is to evaluate the accuracy, significance and relevance of the information in the document and to assess the health and environmental risks from exposure to the chemical. A summary and recommendations for further research and improved safety aspects are also required. The composition of the Task Group is dictated by the range of expertise required for the subject of the meeting and by the need for a balanced geographical distribution.

EHC PREPARATION FLOW CHART

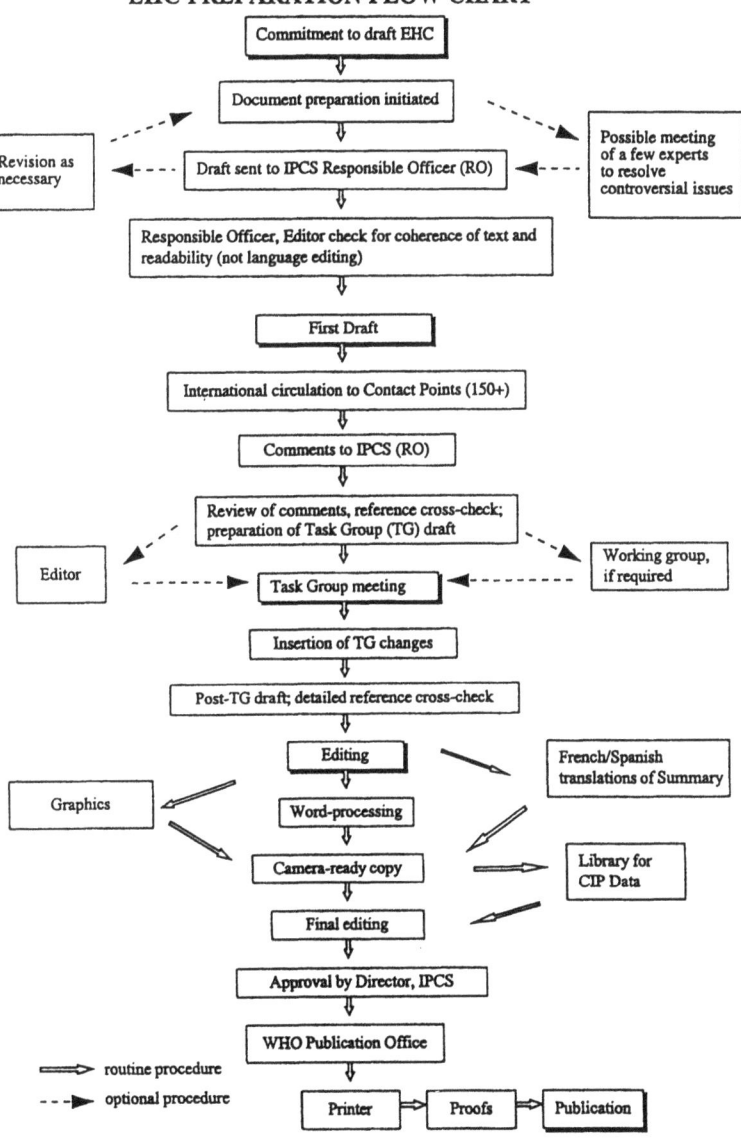

EHC 228: Assessment of Risk from Essential Trace Elements

The three cooperating organizations of the IPCS recognize the important role played by nongovernmental organizations. Representatives from relevant national and international associations may be invited to join the Task Group as observers. Although observers may provide a valuable contribution to the process, they can only speak at the invitation of the Chairperson. Observers do not participate in the final evaluation of the chemical; this is the sole responsibility of the Task Group members. When the Task Group considers it to be appropriate, it may meet *in camera*.

All individuals who as authors, consultants or advisers participate in the preparation of the EHC monograph must, in addition to serving in their personal capacity as scientists, inform the RO if at any time a conflict of interest, whether actual or potential, could be perceived in their work. They are required to sign a conflict of interest statement. Such a procedure ensures the transparency and probity of the process.

When the Task Group has completed its review and the RO is satisfied as to the scientific correctness and completeness of the document, it then goes for language editing, reference checking and preparation of camera-ready copy. After approval by the Director, IPCS, the monograph is submitted to the WHO Office of Publications for printing. At this time a copy of the final draft is sent to the Chairperson and Rapporteur of the Task Group to check for any errors.

It is accepted that the following criteria should initiate the updating of an EHC monograph: new data are available that would substantially change the evaluation; there is public concern for health or environmental effects of the agent because of greater exposure; an appreciable time period has elapsed since the last evaluation.

All Participating Institutions are informed, through the EHC progress report, of the authors and institutions proposed for the drafting of the documents. A comprehensive file of all comments received on drafts of each EHC monograph is maintained and is available on request. The Chairpersons of Task Groups are briefed before each meeting on their role and responsibility in ensuring that these rules are followed.

IPCS WORKING GROUP ON PRINCIPLES AND METHODS FOR THE ASSESSMENT OF RISK FROM ESSENTIAL TRACE ELEMENTS

April 27 – May 1, 1998

Members

Professor P.J. Aggett, Lancashire Postgraduate School of Medicine and Health, University of Central Lancashire, Preston, United Kingdom

Dr R. Goyer, Chapel Hill, NC, USA *(Rapporteur)*

Dr A. Langley, South Australian Health Commission, Adelaide, Australia *(Chairman)*

Dr K. Mahaffey, National Center for Environmental Assessment, US Environmental Protection Agency, Washington DC, USA

Professor M.R. Moore, National Research Centre for Environmental Toxicology, University of Queensland, Coopers Plains, Queensland, Australia

Professor G. Nordberg, Department of Environmental Medicine, University of Umea, Umea, Sweden

Dr S. Olin, International Life Sciences Institute, Risk Science Institute, Washington DC, USA

Dr M. Olivares, Institute of Nutrition and Food Technology, University of Chile, Santiago, Chile

Professor A. Oskarsson, Department of Food Hygiene, School of Veterinary Medicine, Swedish University of Agricultural Sciences, Uppsala, Sweden

Dr M. Ruz, Centre for Human Nutrition, Faculty of Medicine, University of Chile, Santiago, Chile

Dr B. Sandstrom, Research Department of Human Nutrition, Royal Veterinary and Agricultural University, Copenhagen, Denmark

Dr R. Uauy, Institute of Nutrition and Food Technology, University of Chile, Santiago, Chile

Observers and representatives of nongovernmental organizations

Dr J.R. Coughlin *(representing European Centre for Ecotoxicology and Toxicology of Chemicals),* Newport Coast, CA, USA

Dr R. Gaunt *(representing International Commission on Metals in Environment)* Rio Tinto, Bristol, United Kingdom

Secretariat

Dr R. Belmar, Division of Environmental Health, Ministry of Health, Santiago, Chile

Dr G.C. Becking, Kingston, Ontario, Canada

Dr M. Younes, International Programme on Chemical Safety, World Health Organization, Geneva, Switzerland *(Secretary)*

IPCS TASK GROUP ON PRINCIPLES AND METHODS FOR THE ASSESSMENT OF RISK FROM ESSENTIAL TRACE ELEMENTS

26 February - 2 March 2001

Members

Dr C. Abernathy, Office of Water, US Environmental Protection Agency, Washington, DC, USA (*Chairman*)

Professor P.J. Aggett, Lancashire Postgraduate School of Medicine and Health, University of Central Lancashire, Preston, United Kingdom

Dr J. Alexander, Department of Environmental Medicine, National Institute of Public Health, Torshov, Oslo, Norway

Dr M. Araya, Human Nutrition/Clinical Nutrition, National Institute of Nutrition (INTA), Santiago, Chile (*Vice-Chairman*)

Mr P. Callan, Health Advisory Section, National Health and Medical Research Council, Canberra, ACT, Australia (*Rapporteur*)

Dr B.H. Chen, Department of Environmental Health, School of Public Health, Shanghai Medical University, Shanghai, People's Republic of China

Dr R.A. Goyer, Chapel Hill, NC, USA

Dr M.R. L'Abbé, Nutrition Research Section, Bureau of Nutritional Sciences, Health Protection Branch, Health Canada, Banting Research Centre, Tunney's Pasture, Ottawa, Ontario, Canada

Professor G. Nordberg, Department of Environmental Medicine, Umea University, Umea, Sweden

Dr M. Olivares, Institute of Nutrition and Food Technology (INTA), University of Chile, Santiago, Chile

Professor A. Oskarsson, Department of Pharmacology and Toxicology, Swedish University of Agricultural Sciences, Uppsala, Sweden

Dr S. Pavittranon, National Institute of Health, Department of Medical Sciences, Ministry of Public Health, Nonthaburi, Thailand

Dr J.R. Turnlund, US Department of Agriculture, Western Human Nutrition Research Center, San Francisco, CA, USA

Observers

Dr S. Baker, Environmental Program, International Copper Association Ltd., New York, USA (*Representing the International Council on Metals and the Environment*)

Mr G. Lagos Cruz-Coke, Centre of Mineral and Metallurgic Investigation (CIMM), Vitacura, Santiago, Chile

Secretariat

Dr G.C. Becking, Kingston, Ontario, Canada

Dr R. Belmar, Ministry of Health, Santiago, Chile

Dr M. Younes, International Programme on Chemical Safety, World Health Organization, Geneva, Switzerland (*Secretary*)

PRINCIPLES AND METHODS FOR THE ASSESSMENT OF RISK FROM ESSENTIAL TRACE ELEMENTS

A WHO Task Group on "Principles and methods for the assessment of risks from exposure to essential trace elements" met in Marbella, Chile, from 26 February to 2 March 2001. The participants were welcomed on behalf of the Government of Chile by Dr R. Belmar, Cabinet Ministry of Health. The meeting was opened by Dr M. Younes, on behalf of the Coordinator, IPCS and the three cooperating organizations (UNEP/ILO/WHO). In his remarks, Dr Younes thanked the Ministry of Health of Chile for financial support and assistance in organizing the Task Group, as well as an earlier Working Group, and also the Office of Water, US Environmental Protection Agency, for financial support for the development of this monograph. The Task Group reviewed and revised the draft monograph, and developed a series of scientific principles and a conceptual framework for the assessment of risks from exposure to essential trace elements.

The first draft of this monograph, which was reviewed by an IPCS Working Group in April 1998, was prepared by Dr R. Goyer (University of Western Ontario, Canada) with the generous support of the South Australian Health Commission. Based on the discussions of the Working Group, recent scientific data, and comments from the IPCS Contact Points, a Task Group draft was prepared by Dr G.C. Becking (Kingston, Canada) with the assistance of Dr Goyer.

Dr M. Younes and Dr P.G. Jenkins (IPCS Central Unit) were responsible for the technical content and technical editing, respectively, of this monograph.

The efforts of all who helped in the preparation and finalization of this publication are gratefully acknowledged.

ABBREVIATIONS

ADI	acceptable daily intake
AROI	acceptable range of oral intake
BMD	benchmark dose
CI	confidence interval
ETE	essential trace element
LOAEL	lowest-observed-adverse-effect level
NOAEL	no-observed-adverse-effect level
PTDI	provisional tolerable daily intake
PTWI	provisional tolerable weekly intake
RDA	recommended dietary allowance
RfD	reference dose
SD	standard deviation
SF	safety factor
SRPMI	safe range of population mean intake
TDI	tolerable daily intake
TI	tolerable intake
TWI	tolerable weekly intake
UF	uncertainty factor

1. SUMMARY

The risk assessment approach described in this monograph applies only to essential trace elements (ETEs) involved in human health and not to non-essential elements. The monograph is designed to give methods that provide a framework for analysing the boundaries between deficient and excess oral intakes of ETEs. Application of the principles described in this monograph involves a multidisciplinary scientific assessment, using data on required nutritive intakes, deficiency and excess exposure.

This monograph focusses on the concepts of the acceptable range of oral intake (AROI). The AROI is designed to limit deficient and excess intakes in healthy populations and is set for different age-sex groups and physiological states such as pregnancy and lactation. To facilitate comparisons, AROIs are discussed in relation to other risk assessment approaches.

Homeostatic mechanisms involve regulation of absorption and excretion and tissue retention, which enable adaptation to varying nutrient intakes. These mechanisms provide for an optimal systemic supply for the performance of essential functions and must be considered in establishing an AROI. The impact of other factors, such as chemical form, dietary characteristics and interactions amongst ETEs, are also critical in determining the AROI for ETEs.

When ETE intakes are above or below the boundaries of the AROI, the capacity of the homeostatic mechanisms is exceeded and the probability and severity of adverse effects increase. The homeostatic model was used to establish the AROI and is illustrated with examples and a series of theoretical curves.

The process begins with the selection of the database for a particular ETE. A weight-of-evidence approach is then used for hazard identification, selecting relevant end-points of deficient and excess exposures. Next, the probability of risk and the severity of various effects are quantified and critical effects are selected. The AROI is then established by balancing end-points of comparable health significance. At this time, the exposure assessment is conducted. Finally, a risk characterization enumerating the strengths and weaknesses of the databases is performed, integrating the AROI and exposure assessment.

2. INTRODUCTION

2.1 Scope and purpose

The purpose of this monograph is to develop the scientific principles that support the concept of an "acceptable range of oral intake" (AROI), which uses a "homeostatic model" for determining the range of dietary intakes for essential trace elements (ETEs) that meet the nutritional requirements of a healthy population and avoid excess intakes. Although it includes examples, this monograph is not a compendium of assessments on ETEs, nor is it a textbook detailing the scientific basis of risk assessment or the derivation of dietary reference intakes.

The principles and methods developed in this monograph are intended for ETEs and are not necessarily applicable to toxic non-essential elements or other chemicals. Trace elements currently regarded by the World Health Organization as essential for human health are iron (WHO, 1988), zinc, copper, chromium, iodine, cobalt, molybdenum and selenium (WHO, 1996).

A second group of elements (silicon, manganese, nickel, boron and vanadium), which might have some beneficial effects and which are classified by WHO as probably essential for humans (WHO, 1996), are not considered in this monograph. If any one of these, or other elements, becomes accepted as essential for humans and quantitative requirements are established, then the approaches devised in this monograph should be applicable for setting an AROI for these elements.

The methodology presented in this monograph recognizes the importance of:

- variability of the efficiency of intestinal uptake and transfer of the ETE arising from the composition of the diet and food matrix containing the ETE;

- variability in intake and kinetics arising from age, gender, physiological conditions and nutritional status;

- person-to-person variability of unknown origin;

- short-term exposures during critical periods that greatly alter the risk and nature of adverse effects, e.g., developmental effects in fetuses, infants and young children;

- consideration of whether or not the adverse effects are fully reversible following increases or decreases in oral intake of ETEs;

- recognition that dietary/food intake is only part of oral intake. Oral intake also includes intake from water and beverages, dietary supplements and a fraction of inhalation exposures that become orally available after having been transported via the mucillary transport system and swallowed.

Excluded from consideration are:

- carcinogenicity of ETEs;

- metals, such as lead, mercury and cadmium, that are not known to provide any essential or potentially beneficial health effect at any level of exposure;

- ETEs used for pharmaco-therapeutic purposes;

- ecotoxicity of essential trace elements.

The need to develop methodology for assessing the toxicity of ETEs arose from an awareness that, for some ETEs, the margin between individual and population requirements and the estimate of the tolerable intake (TI) may be very small, and in some instances these values may overlap among individuals and populations. There are several reasons why these difficulties have occurred. These include differences in methodologies between nutritionists and toxicologists, lack of interaction between the two groups, and lack of oversight and co-ordination by different advisory and regulatory bodies. Furthermore, recommended dietary allowances (RDAs) and TIs are determined by

Introduction

conceptually different approaches. Toxicologists customarily think in terms of high intakes, the risk of toxicity, and application of uncertainty factors, at least for non-cancer endpoints, whereas nutritionists are primarily concerned with avoiding inadequate intakes and the risk of deficiency.

The difficulties inherent in this task have been recognized previously. A workshop sponsored by the US Environmental Protection Agency, the Agency for Toxic Substances and Disease Registry, and the International Life Sciences Institute's Risk Science Institute (held in March 1992) reviewed the problems inherent in the assessment of risk from human exposure to low and high intakes of ETEs, and identified a number of topics that had been inadequately considered (Mertz et al., 1994). Similarly, a Nordic Working Group on Food and Nutrition and the Nordic Working Group on Food Toxicology have prepared a report "Risk evaluation of essential trace elements - essential versus toxic levels of intake" (Oskarsson, 1995), and a conference on "Risk assessment for essential trace elements - contrasting essentiality and toxicity" was held in Stockholm in May 1992 (Nordberg & Skerfving, 1993). More recently concepts and progress in setting intake guidelines for ETEs have been reviewed (Mertz, 1998; Olin, 1998; Sandström, 1998). In addition, the Food & Nutrition Board (FNB) of the United States National Academy of Sciences (IOM, 2001) has developed a risk assessment model for establishing "upper intake levels for nutrients" which recognizes the possible benefits of intakes above RDAs, the narrow margins between desirable and undesirable intakes for many ETEs, and the need to ensure that advice from toxicologists and nutritionists is compatible. The European Union Scientific Committee on Food has adopted a report that deals with the development of "tolerable upper intake levels" for vitamins and minerals (SCF, 2000).

2.2 Criteria for essentiality of trace elements

The criteria for identifying nutritionally ETEs have evolved over the past fifty years and may be expected to expand as the result of future research. The traditional criteria for essentiality for human health are that absence or deficiency of the element from the diet produces either functional or structural abnormalities and that the abnormalities are related to, or a consequence of, specific biochemical changes that can be reversed by the presence of the essential metal (WHO, 1996).

End-points used in establishing essentiality of trace elements in experimental animals are impairment of growth and development, neurological effects, inefficient reproduction, loss of tissue integrity, and defects in physiological and biochemical functions. To establish such criteria for particular elements requires an insight of their biological roles, sensitive methods to detect subtle effects, and accurate instrumentation to measure trace amounts of the ETEs (Mertz, 1993).

2.2.1 *Essentiality and homeostatic mechanisms*

ETEs have homeostatic mechanisms involving regulation of absorption and excretion and tissue retention, which enable adaptation to varying nutrient intakes to ensure a safe and optimum systemic supply for the performance of essential functions (section 4.1). There are specific homeostatic mechanisms for each ETE. The possibility that within populations, the efficiency of homeostasis may vary is considered in section 4.1. However, identification of the prevalence of any variation would require the study of large populations. Many characteristic interactions of ETEs (e.g., Zn/Cu; Zn/Fe) are described in section 4.7.

Risk assessments become more certain when the homeostatic mechanisms for each ETE are considered. Known defects in homeostasis, either secondary to disease or genetically based, require consideration in the risk assessment process. However, their inclusion in setting public health guidelines on food safety needs to be considered on a case-by-case basis.

2.3 Terminology

Terms and definitions cited in this document are based on the reports cited above, as well as the IPCS Environmental Health Criteria 170 and 210 (IPCS, 1994, 1999) and "Trace elements in human nutrition and health" (WHO, 1996). Although the terminology and definitions are contained in many other reports, they are presented again as a basis for their use in this monograph.

Introduction

2.3.1 Definitions relating to individual and population requirements for ETEs

The term 'population' refers to a group that is homogenous in terms of age, sex and other characteristics believed to affect requirement (WHO, 1996). In developing AROIs, the term population does not refer to geographically or culturally defined groups or to groups with genetic abnormalities in the metabolism of ETEs.

2.3.1.1 Factorial estimation of nutrient requirement

A starting point in defining nutritional requirements is the use of factorial estimates of nutritional need. The "factorial model" is based on the minimum requirement of the nutrient for replacement of losses from excretion and utilization at low intakes without reducing body stores and is usually sufficient for prevention of clinical deficiency in adults. Factorial methods are used only as a first approximation to the assessment of individual requirements or when functional, clinical or biochemical criteria of adequacy have not been established (WHO, 1996).

2.3.1.2 Requirements for the individual

Requirement for the individual, as stated in WHO (1996), is the lowest continuing level of nutrient intake that, at a specified efficiency of utilization, will maintain the defined level of nutriture in the individual. For nutritionally ETEs, the defined level of nutriture may concern a basal requirement or a normative requirement or both. The basal requirement is the level of intake needed to prevent pathologically relevant and clinically detectable signs of impaired function attributable to inadequacy of the nutrient. The normative requirement refers to the level of intake that serves to maintain a level of tissue storage or other reserve that is judged to be desirable. The difference between intakes meeting the basal requirement and the normative requirement represents the protective buffer provided by systemic stores and homeostatic adaptations when intakes are low. Thus when intakes are below the estimated normative requirement, mobilization of stores and other adaptive phenomena would be evidence of "deficiency". Below the basal level, homeostatic adaptation is more likely to be inadequate, and metabolic and other disturbances would be expected.

2.3.1.3 Dietary reference intakes, population reference intakes, reference nutrient intakes, recommended dietary allowance, and safe range of population mean intake

Many different terms, definitions and values are used by various countries and organizations (European Union, North America and World Health Organization) in developing recommendations for dietary intakes of ETEs. For example, new terms have been developed such as the dietary reference intake (DRI) (IOM, 2001) and by European Union (SCF, 2000). The definitions have similarities but there are often subtle differences in their meaning and application. There is need to harmonize universally the terms and definitions used to describe recommended dietary intakes, including the upper level of intake based on toxicological data.

Most earlier reports on recommended intakes of essential elements have provided estimates of the requirements of individuals, and the "recommended" dietary intake that would be expected to meet the needs of the majority (97.5%) of a defined population has been defined as the average dietary requirement plus 2 standard deviations (SD). Thus, for an individual consuming this amount of element there would be a very low probability of the requirement not being met. WHO (1996) is concerned with population (group) mean intakes rather than intakes of individuals. The lower limit of population mean intake, i.e., the "safe range of population mean intake" (SRPMI), is set so that very few individuals in the population (group) would be expected to have intakes below their requirement, i.e., the estimates of average individual requirement plus 2 standard deviations. The basic concept of the SRPMI is illustrated in Fig. 1 (WHO, 1996).

The variability in usual intakes within a population group is usually larger than estimates of variability of requirements, and it has been demonstrated empirically that the evaluation of the prevalence of inadequate intakes is relatively insensitive to the variability in estimates of the requirements (WHO, 1996).

Introduction

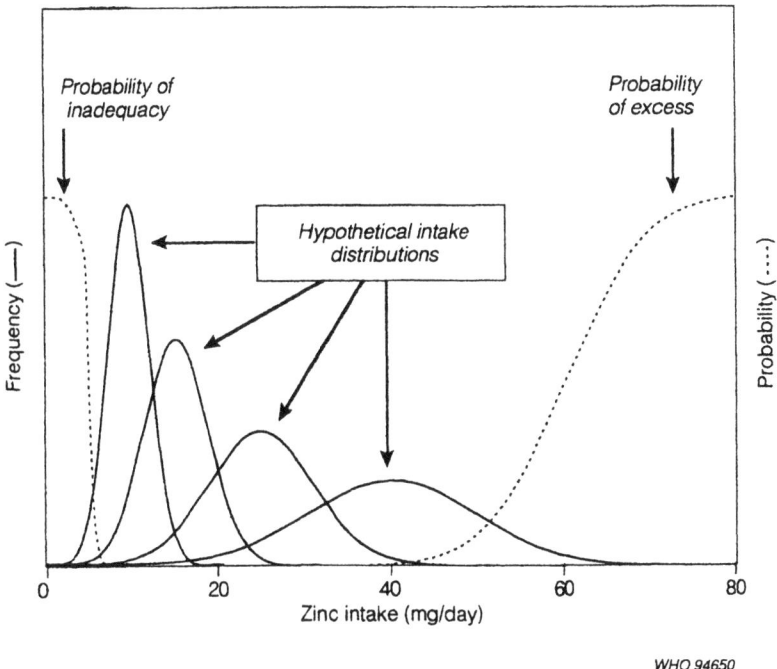

Fig. 1. The concept of the safe range of population mean intakes

The diagram shows the risk curves for the probability of inadequacy of intake and of excess of intake (risk to individual), together with a series of intake distributions, all of which would be associated with a low prevalence of effects of either inadequate or excess intake. All these intake distributions would be characterized as falling within the safe range of population mean intakes. The diagram is based on the zinc intakes of young adult men consuming a diet of moderate zinc availability.

2.3.2 Toxicological terms

2.3.2.1 Acceptable daily intake, tolerable intake, tolerable upper intake level

Many terms and definitions have been proposed for the health-based guidance values developed from the dose–response relationships in toxicological studies. These include: acceptable daily intake (ADI) (IPCS, 1987); tolerable intake (TI), which may be daily (TDI) or weekly (TWI) (IPCS, 1994); provisional tolerable weekly (daily) intake (PTW(D)I) (IPCS, 1987); tolerable upper intake level (UL) (SCF, 2000; IOM, 2001). ADI and TDI are estimates of the amount of a substance that can be ingested daily over a lifetime without appreciable risk. The ADI is applied to estimates for food additives, whereas TDI is used for those relating to contaminants. The UL is the maximum level of daily intake of a nutrient judged to be unlikely to pose a risk of adverse health effects to humans.

2.3.2.2 Reference dose

The US Environmental Protection Agency has replaced the ADI and TDI with the single term, reference dose (RfD), which is defined as an estimate (with uncertainty spanning perhaps an order of magnitude) of a daily exposure for the human population (including sensitive subgroups) that is likely to be without an appreciable risk of deleterious effects during a lifetime. The term RfD is intended to avoid any implication that exposure to the chemical is completely "safe" or "acceptable", as may be implied by use of the term ADI (Dourson, 1994). As for the ADI/TDI, the RfD assumes that zero exposure to the element of concern is without risk. For ETEs, this is not an appropriate default position.

2.3.3 Principles underlying derivation of nutrient requirements and tolerable intakes

The major differences between the assumptions underlying derivation of nutrient requirements (e.g., RDAs) and TIs are highlighted in Table 1, expanding upon the points raised by Bowman & Risher (1994). These differences must be considered in determining for ETEs scientifically based assessments that are broadly protective for both low and high exposures. Principles for identifying nutrient requirements of ETEs have been reviewed in WHO (1996). Principles

Introduction

Table 1. Comparison of principles underlying derivation of nutrient requirements and tolerable intakes (TIs) for ETEs[a]

Principle	Nutrient requirements	Toxicological limits
Human exposure	only presumed sources are food and water	all sources (TI) oral only (RfD and ADI)
Use of data	bioavailability, nutrient and dietary interactions all considered	only toxicity usually considered
Population addressed and protected	normally developed for specific age-sex groups and physiological states in general population	usually all healthy groups of consumers over 3 months of age
Clinical significance	deficiency states can lead to clinical effects or inadequate stores	adverse end-point chosen often with limited information on clinical significance

[a] These principles are discussed more fully in the appropriate sections of the text.

for evaluating excess exposures from ETEs have been summarized in recent conferences (Mertz et al., 1994; Oskarsson, 1995; IOM, 2001), but there has been much less research involved in identifying TIs for ETEs than for the characterization of adverse health effects of non-essential metals.

For ETEs, the use of diet as the only source of exposure considered for a RDA is not too critical, since food makes by far the major contribution to exposure from an ETE. In some instances (such as copper) drinking-water can be a significant source (IPCS, 1998).

2.3.4 Approaches to define a threshold dose

Data used to determine a TI are rarely absolutely certain and complete, so compensatory adjustments have to be made. One approach is to use uncertainty factors (UFs) which are devised to reduce experimentally or clinically identified toxicological thresholds (e.g., NOAEL, LOAEL) to account for scientific uncertainties including inadequacies in the scientific database as well as variability.

An alternative method, generally called the benchmark dose approach, is to analyse the dose–response curve, including the confidence around the central estimate, thereby deriving a more precise estimation based on all the available data (see Fig. 2).

2.3.5 Characteristics of uncertainty factors

Uncertainty factors (UF) are applied to a no-observed-adverse-effect level (NOAEL) or lowest-observed-adverse-effect level (LOAEL) to derive an ADI, TDI or RfD. Uncertainty or safety factors are determined on the basis of the adequacy and quality of the overall database available.

The traditional approach to determining an uncertainty factor is to identify the individual factors influencing the uncertainty. These factors should represent the adequacy of the pivotal study, interspecies extrapolation, differences in susceptibility of individuals in the human population, nature of toxicity, and adequacy of the overall database, taking into account high-dose to low-dose extrapolations and extrapolations from short-term to chronic effects (Younes et al., 1998). The product of single factors is determined and used for calculating the ADI, TI, or RfD from the observed NOAEL or LOAEL:

$$TDI = \frac{NOAEL \text{ or } LOAEL}{\text{Total product of UFs}}$$

A factor of 100 is generally considered appropriate as a default factor for chronic animal exposures studies (IPCS, 1987). The value of 100 has been regarded to comprise two factors of 10, to allow for inter-species extrapolation and inter-individual (within species) variations. In instances of one, two or three areas of uncertainty, the UF becomes 10, 100 or 1000, respectively. This approach was developed for providing TDIs for toxic metals with non-carcinogenic end-points, which are generally assumed to be threshold events.

Beck et al. (1995) suggested that the value of 10 may overestimate differences between subchronic and chronic NOAEL and LOAEL levels, so that UFs of 3, 5 or 7 may be the most appropriate. Data from Pieters et al. (1998) provide support for the retention of a UF of 10.

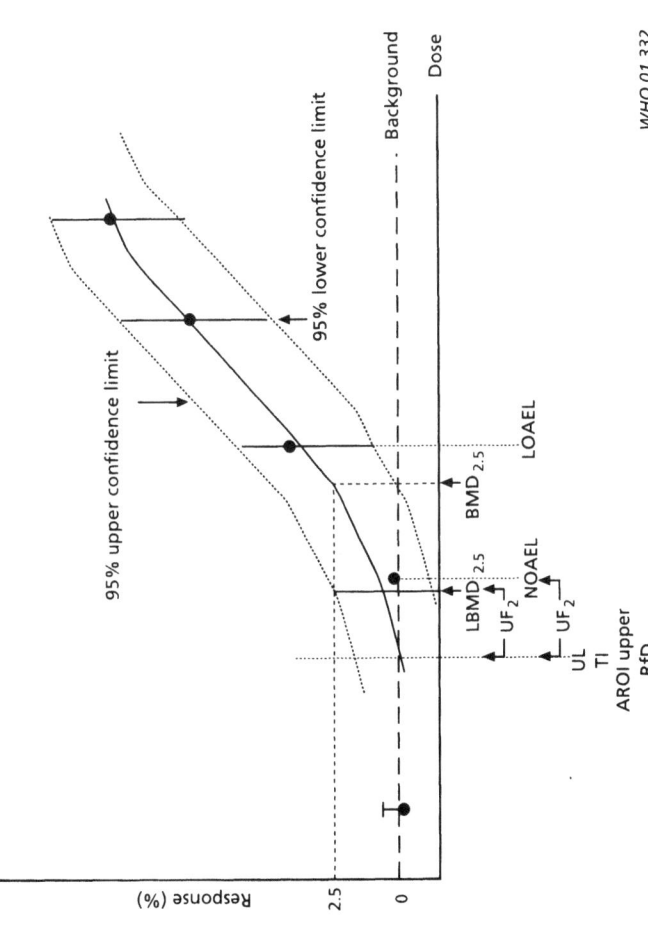

Fig. 2. Theoretical representation of the lower part of the dose–response curve for a minimal adverse effect in a sensitive population with the upper 95% of confidence limit of the response

95% CI of background estimate is also indicated. $BMD_{2.5}$ is the benchmark dose where 2.5% of the individuals experience an adverse effect. $LBMD_{2.5}$ is the lower 95% CI of the $BMD_{2.6}$ i.e. where no more than 2.5% of the individuals experience the minimal adverse effect (estimated with 95% certainty). NOAEL is the no-observed-adverse-effect level. UF1 is the uncertainty factor applied to the NOAEL when deriving TI of UL (upper tolerable level), and UF2 is the uncertainty factor applied to $LBMD_{2.5}$ when deriving the upper bound of the AROI. BMD has been referred to in earlier publications as "effective dose" (ED) while LBMD was termed "benchmark dose" (BD) (Crump, 1984; IPCS, 1994).

However, the authors prefer to use dose–response modelling to avoid use of an NOAEL or LOAEL. On the other hand, differences in individual susceptibility may warrant a much larger UF than 10.

A refinement of using uncertainty factors is that of subdividing the two default factors of 10 to allow for any known toxicodynamic and toxicokinetic variability (IPCS, 1994). However, such data are often lacking and the traditional UF approach may be the only option. Nevertheless, research efforts are underway to identify means for using data-derived UFs (Dourson et al., 1996). Guidance on the use of factors derived from actual data (termed "adjustment factors") has been developed by the IPCS (IPCS, 1999).

The selection of UFs is a critical step in determining a TDI for ETEs. The use of large UFs for an ETE could increase the risk of nutritional deficiency. Therefore, selection of appropriate UFs for ETEs must consider potential effects in both directions, nutritional deficiency and toxicity. Human data are generally available for ETEs and often describes the variability between individuals. Thus, UFs of less than 10 may be used, as has been done for zinc (Cantilli et al., 1994).

2.3.6 Estimating TI from dose–response curve for critical effect

The entire dose–response curve and the variation in response within the studied population are not considered when a NOAEL/LOAEL is used for establishing the TI. A dose–response curve can provide more precise estimation of the confidence levels around the estimate, and other information about the uncertainties of the data.

Approaches using more of the data from the dose–response curve have been used in criteria documents for non-essential toxic metals, e.g., methylmercury (IPCS, 1990) and cadmium (IPCS, 1992). For these two substances the upper confidence limit around the dose–response curve for the critical effect was used to assure safety.

One approach to dealing with dose–response information is the benchmark dose approach (Crump, 1984) (see Fig. 2, which was also described in IPCS, 1994). It is defined by IPCS (1994) as: "The lower

Introduction

confidence limit [95% statistical lower bound] of the dose that produces a small increase in the level of adverse effects, (e.g., 5 or 10%), to which uncertainty factors can be applied to develop a tolerable intake." It is different from the NOAEL/LOAEL approach in that it is derived from the entire dose–response curve. The magnitude of the confidence limits provides an indication of the power of the study and quality of the data.

Uncertainty factors are generally applied as part of the benchmark dose approach. A UF > 1 is often applied to account for person-to-person variability, although, if the most sensitive group of the population is studied, a UF of 1 may be used.

3. THE ACCEPTABLE RANGE OF ORAL INTAKE FOR AN ESSENTIAL TRACE ELEMENT

3.1 Definition of an AROI

The acceptable range of oral intake (AROI) for an ETE is represented by a trough in the U-shaped dose–response curve spanning requirements for essentiality to toxic levels, as shown in Fig. 3. The normal physiological range is between points A and B and is identified as the AROI. The lower margin of AROI (point A) is usually equivalent to the RDA, i.e., the 2.5% of the population under consideration will be at risk of deficiency (in other words, will be at risk of minimal adverse effects). Ideally, the higher margin of AROI (point B) is the $LBMD_{2.5}$ for minimal adverse effects. However, due to sparse data sets and information on homeostasis, the TI or UL may often be used to set the higher margin.

The breadth and location of the trough on the dose–response curve is subject to the variability in populations, as discussed in section 4. Establishing an AROI for an ETE requires balancing the nutritional requirement for a particular element and the potential for a toxic effect from over-exposure. Although the AROI and SRPMI are based on different concepts, one way of assessing whether a population intake falls within the AROI is to use techniques such as the SRPMI described in section 2.3.1.3. The difference in the percentage of the population at risk from the choice of the SRPMI compared to choosing the AROI will be affected by the slope (i.e. shape) of the relevant intake distributions and the slope of the risk of toxicity or deficiency curves.

The figure of 2.5% is based on 2 standard deviations from the means of the distributions for requirements and risks of toxicity. The value of 2.5% might change according to the nature and severity of the effects of concern, the shape of the distribution and the breadth of the AROI. A more detailed description is provided in section 3.2. The toxicity and deficiency will refer to the toxic or deficiency effect (endpoint) of concern rather than overt clinical toxicity or deficiency.

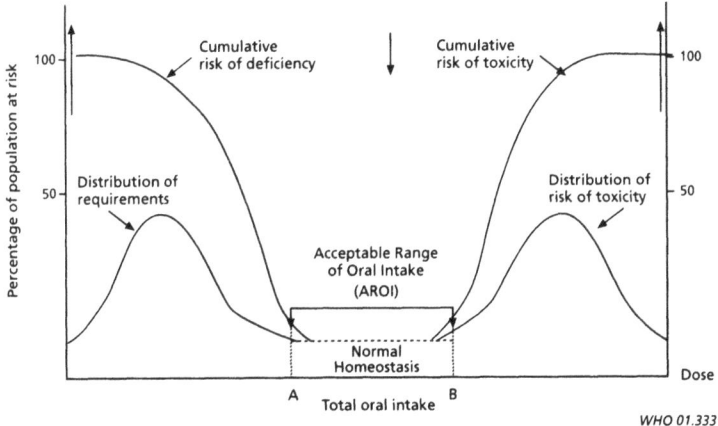

Fig. 3. Percentage of population at risk of deficiency and toxicity effects according to oral intake.

As ETE intakes drop below A (lower limit of AROI where 2.5% of the population under consideration will be at risk of deficiency), an increasing proportion will be at risk of deficiency. At extremely low intakes all subjects will manifest deficiency. As ETE intakes exceed B (where 2.5% of the population under consideration will be at risk of toxicity), a progressively larger proportion of the population will be at risk of toxicity.

3.2 Boundaries of an AROI

It is important to understand that neither the lower nor upper boundary of the AROI is an absolute value below which or above which adverse effects occur. The definition of nutritional requirement has been fixed for a population but there is considerable variability of requirement among individuals. Therefore, at intakes greater than B, the risk of toxicity will increase or the severity of effect noted might increase with dose, but not all individuals will have the same sensitivity at intakes above point B. The same concept holds for intakes lower than A with regard to signs of deficiency.

3.2.1 Lower limit of an AROI

Fig. 4 describes the dose–response curves for the development of deficiency effects when the basal requirements are not met. The curve for the normative requirement is also shown. The mean plus 2 standard deviations of the normative requirement is usually used as the lower limit of the AROI. This requires that there is no overlap with the upper limit of the AROI (see further discussion in section 5).

3.2.2 Upper limit of an AROI

Fig. 2 displays a theoretical benchmark (Gaylor et al., 1998) analysis of a dose–response curve in order to explain how derivations of such boundaries can be performed. In order to derive these points the full data set on which the dose–response curve for toxicity is based needs to be considered. However, the shapes of the toxicity and deficiency curves may not be symmetrical. Homeostatic mechanisms may be overwhelmed, and risks of toxicity increased or decreased depending on the precision in the data set and the confidence limits around the dose–response curve (i.e. with wide (low-precision) or narrow (high precision) confidence limits). If the $BMD_{2.5}$ is to be estimated with high certainty (i.e. if one wishes to be 95% certain not to overestimate the $BMD_{2.5}$), it can be estimated at the 95% upper confidence limit instead of at the mean estimate of the dose–response curve (Fig. 2). This level can be designated the $LBMD_{2.5}$, i.e the lower 95% CI of the $BMD_{2.5}$, where no more than 2.5% of the individuals experience the minimal adverse effect.

Uncertainty factors are generally applied as part of the benchmark dose approach. If the most minimal adverse effect is measured in the most sensitive group, a UF of 1 may be appropriate. However, where data are not available for the most sensitive population group or where there is a need to protect a larger proportion of the population than the benchmark chosen, a UF > 1 is applied. This would also be the case for an ETE that is known to result in less severe but adverse effects below the 95% CI of the $BMD_{2.5}$.

Some of the problems in setting the boundaries of the AROI arise from lack of knowledge of signs or biomarkers of marginal states of deficiency or toxicity. In addition, the rigid application of large uncertainty factors to the NOAEL without concern for bioavailability,

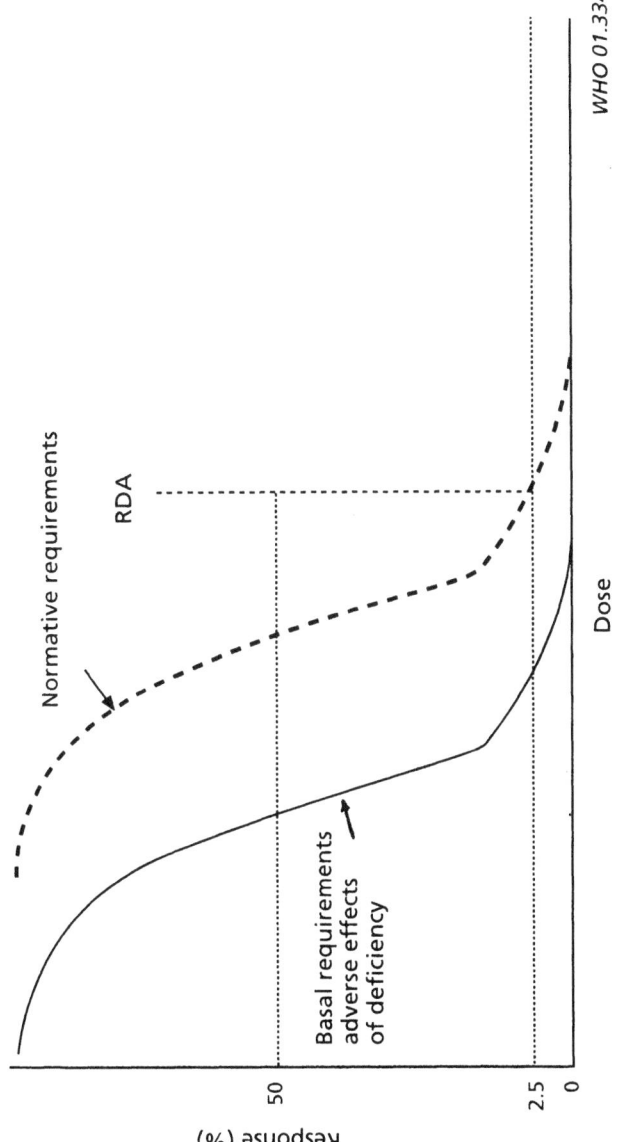

Fig. 4. Dose–response curves for the development of deficiency effects when the basal requirements are not met

nutrient interactions and homeostatic mechanisms can lead to point B being given a lower value than point A in Fig. 3.

As has been pointed out in section 2, some subpopulations may exhibit toxicity at levels below the acceptable range (e.g., Wilson's disease) or deficiency at levels higher than recommended intakes (e.g., acrodermatitis enteropathica). These groups would not be part of the risk assessment considered in this monograph. It may be necessary, nevertheless, to consider these subgroups in risk management. They are described further in section 4.

Although the term AROI is used in this document to facilitate a comparison with the RDA, which only considers dietary intake, the concept of a range of intakes within which homeostasis is maintained can be applied to situations where other routes of exposure are significant.

The concept of SRPMI described in section 2.3.1.3, and more fully in WHO (1996), which is based on observations of mean intakes and their distribution, provides another way of safety assessment. If greater protection from toxicity is deemed necessary, a value different from the $LBMD_{2.5}$ (i.e. lower 95% CI of $BMD_{2.5}$) may be applied depending on the nature and severity of the end-point.

3.3 Comparison of safety evaluations

An AROI is usually specified for particular population groups such as those defined by age, gender or physiological status (e.g., lactation, pregnancy) and defines a range of safe intakes in individuals belonging to the specified group. It requires that the boundaries for excess (see Fig. 2) and the limit for deficiency (see Fig. 4) can be estimated with all possible precision and accuracy. This may be difficult in practice. On the other hand, when sufficient data are available, upper and lower limits can be calculated (e.g., RDA and BMD). Use of these methodologies enables the calculation of risks of deficiency or excess to a defined percentage (e.g., to a maximum of 2.5%). In assessing whether a particular population group under consideration has risks greater than 2.5%, the distribution of intakes has to be compared with the AROI. Since all individuals in such a population group cannot be studied, the assessment will usually be based on measurements of intakes in a representative sample of the group. Mean intake and the distribution of intakes will be estimated, and these numbers will be used to assess whether or not intakes are within the AROI and the likelihood of deficiency and excess. The proportion of a population that can be allowed to fall outside of the AROI will be evaluated in each case and depends on what adverse health effects have been used to define the AROI.

The concept of an AROI is fully consistent with the US Food and Nutrition Board (FNB) model for the determination of dietary reference intakes (DRIs) (IOM, 2001). The European Union's Scientific Committee on Food has also reported on the development of tolerable upper intake levels for vitamins and minerals (SCF, 2000).

4. VARIABILITY OF HUMAN POPULATIONS

This section highlights some of the information on factors that may lead to variable responses to ETE exposures in defined life-stage population groups. These factors include homeostasis, bioavailability, dietary and nutrient interactions, and age-related factors. It is beyond the scope of this monograph to discuss each of these factors in detail. However, one or more of the following references should be consulted for more details on the scientific support for this information: general background information (WHO, 1996; Ziegler & Filer, 1996; IOM, 2001); homeostasis (Anderson, 1996; Pena et al., 1999; Camakaris et al., 1999); bioavailability (Fairweather-Tait & Hurrell, 1996; ILSI, 1997; Schümann et al., 1997); speciation and interactions (Bodwell & Erdan, 1988; Bremner & Beattie, 1995; Telisman, 1995).

4.1 Principles of homeostasis of ETEs in humans

ETEs can be thought of as comprising three groups, namely those that are handled as cations (zinc, iron, copper, manganese, chromium), those handled as anions (molybdenum, iodine, selenium), and those handled as a bio-inorganic complex (e.g. cobalt).

For each category the body has evolved specific mechanisms for the acquisition and retention, storage and excretion of the various elements. For cations those homeostatic mechanisms operate predominantly via the gastrointestinal tract and the liver, and may regulate the uptake and transfer of the metals by the gut (e.g., iron, zinc, copper) or by biliary excretion (copper). For instance, copper absorption decreases from 75% at 0.4 mg/day to 12% at 7.5 mg/day, but the total amount absorbed increases. Homeostasis has been shown by a dose–response curve demonstrating the effect of copper intake on the regulation of copper absorption (Turnlund et al., 1989). Most of the additional copper absorbed is then excreted via the bile (Turnlund et al., 1998). Because these cationic ETEs are chemically reactive, lipophobic and poorly soluble at physiological pH, animals have evolved systems to regulate closely both their amount and activity in the body. Thus for each cationic element there is thought to be a specific chain of carriers in the enterocytes (Gunshin, 1997; Donovan et al., 2000). They are involved in: (i) transfer of the element around the circulation (e.g., transferrin, caeruloplasmin, albumin, transcuprein, metallothionein) (Cox, 1999; Andrews, 1999; McKie et al., 2000; Nordberg & Nordberg, 2000), (ii) their uptake into organs (e.g., transferrin receptors, caeruloplasmin receptors, metallothionein), (iii) their compartmentalization and egress from cells (e.g., possibly the Cu-ATPases involved in Menkes and Wilson's diseases), and (iv) the sequestration of the elements (either storage or detoxification devices in tissues (e.g., apoferritin, metallothioneins)). Although each such chain of control provides an overall selective pathway for its respective element, *in vitro* studies indicate that each step or carrier is not necessarily specific; interactions can occur with other metals at several sites. Nevertheless, each sequence achieves an effective delivery of its respective ETE in appropriate quantities to appropriate functional or storage sites.

By no means have all the (protein) carriers involved been identified, but some regulatory mechanisms have been identified for those that have been characterized and such information encourages confidence that other carriers (e.g., the enterocytic zinc uptake mechanism which is defective in acrodermatitis enteropathica) will be found (Cousins & McMahon, 2000) and that the regulatory mechanisms of their expression will be characterized (Liuzzi et al., 2001). Scenarios for the events of carrier mechanisms and biokinetics in homeostasis can be induced from our current insight of carrier mechanisms and biokinetics, but definitive evidence for much of this is not yet available for humans.

Homeostasis of the cationic ETEs results from the modifications of several of the stages in the elements' chain, but the critical primary control point in limiting excessive accumulation differs between elements. For all the elements the initial adaptation is a down-regulation of the enterocytic uptake mechanisms. For iron the principal homeostatic control occurs by the induction in the enterocyte of apoferritin, which sequesters the metal and prevents its transfer into the body (i.e. a "mucosal block") (Conrad, 1993). In contrast the body burden of zinc is primarily achieved by absorption from and excretion (pancreatic) into the small intestine (Jackson et al., 1984). The control of copper body load is by changes in the efficiency of absorption and biliary excretion (Turnlund et al., 1989; 1998). Additional insight of the metabolic defects in Wilson's and Menkes diseases has improved our understanding of copper homeostasis and prevention of excess accumulation of copper. In healthy individuals, when zinc burdens exceed the capacity of these primary mechanisms, an enterocytic "mucosal block" based on induced metallothionein develops.

The anionic ETEs are more water-soluble and are less reactive with N, S, P, O and OH groups than are cationic ETEs. The systemic acquisition of these elements appears to be much less regulated than it is for cationic ETEs as they are absorbed very efficiently, usually > 70%; their subsequent control, compartmentalization and excretion is managed by manipulation of their oxidation and methylation states and the total body burden is regulated by renal excretion. These processes are best understood for iodine, but the regulation of the enzymes and mechanisms involved are not well characterized. This is the case also for selenium, although characteristic excretion forms of reduced selenium are known. Molybdenum is very efficiently absorbed (> 80%) and the excess is efficiently excreted via the kidneys (Turnlund et al., 1995), but the mechanisms of control are not well understood.

Cobalt is a highly reactive element with several oxidation states. In *in vitro* systems it can effectively compete with many other cationic ETEs and it is conceivable, therefore, that the physiological role for this metal as the highly regulated form in cobalamin has evolved to avoid these problems. There is no evidence that humans require inorganic cobalt.

The development of methodology to identify and measure biomarkers of exposure and effect based on early homeostatic adaptation to inappropriate high intakes of ETEs is being actively pursued.

4.2 Bioavailability

The bioavailability of a nutrient relates to its absorption and may be defined as its accessibility to normal metabolic and physiological processes (SCF, 2000). The bioavailability of trace elements may vary considerably, depending on a number of factors such as food source or dietary matrix, oral intake, chemical form or species of the ETE, nutritional state (deficiency versus excess), age, gender, physiological state, pathological conditions, and interactions with other substances. It is likely that most of these factors have a role in bioavailability for each of the nutritionally essential trace elements. Bioavailability factors are more frequently incorporated in derivation of RDAs than in assessment of toxicity, particularly release of essential elements from food during digestion and absorption efficiency (Bowman & Risher, 1994). However, improved understanding of the factors that affect bioavailability of ETEs provides opportunity to include them in the risk assessment process.

4.2.1 Bioavailability and utilization

The principal variables influencing ETE bioavailability are summarized in Table 2. The most important factor is nutritional status, which influences adaptive processes or biokinetics in response to deficiency or excess. These include absorption, transport, metabolism, excretion and storage of the element, influence of age and gender, pregnancy and lactation, interactions with other elements and chemical speciation. Such factors should be accounted for in determining the AROI.

4.3 Age-related variables

4.3.1 In utero

ETEs are critical for the normal development and growth of the embryo and fetus. Brain development is particularly sensitive to deficiencies of ETEs. For example, zinc is essential for development of the neural tube during embryonic life and differentiation of the brain during the fetal phase of development (Prasad, 1998). Animal studies have shown that deprivation of zinc during gestation may result in a variety of malformations of the nervous system (Warkany & Petering, 1972). Similarly, copper, iron and other ETEs are essential for intrauterine growth and development. During the third trimester, the fetus must accumulate stores of some ETEs (i.e. zinc, copper, iron) for the immediate post-delivery period (Yip & Dallman, 1996; Allen, 1997; IPCS, 1998). If gestation is shortened and birth is premature, there is a failure to accumulate adequate stores of ETEs by the fetus, which may result in deficiencies during the post-natal period.

Table 2. Physiological and dietary variables influencing trace element utilization (from: WHO, 1996)

A. Intrinsic (physiological) variables

1. *Absorptive processes*

   a) *Developmental changes*:

   i) Infancy: immediate postnatal absorption poorly regulated (e.g., of chromium, iron, and zinc) until homeostatic regulatory mechanisms become established with increasing gut maturity

   ii) The elderly: possible decline in efficiency of absorption of copper and zinc

   b) *Homeostatic regulation*:

   adaptation to low trace-element status or high demand (e.g., during pregnancy) by modifying activity/concentration of receptors involved in uptake from gastrointestinal tract (applicable to iron, chromium, copper, manganese, zinc, but probably not to iodine or selenium)

   relationship of intraluminal soluble content of element to proportional saturation of receptors involved in absorption (marked influence on zinc utilization)

2. *Metabolic/functional interactions*

   interdependence of elements in processes involved in storage and metabolism (copper and iron in catecholamine metabolism; selenium in iodine utilization; zinc in protein synthesis/degradation)

   metabolic interrelationships enhancing element loss or reducing mobility of stored element (e.g., tissue anabolism sequestering zinc; physical activity promoting chromium loss, tissue injury promoting skeletal zinc loss)

   metabolic interrelationships enhancing release of stored element (e.g., low calcium promoting skeletal zinc release; tissue catabolism promoting zinc redistribution)

B. Extrinsic (dietary) variables

Solubility and molecular dimensions of trace-element-bearing species within food, digesta and gut lumen influencing mucosal uptake (e.g., non-available iron oxalates, copper sulfides, trace element silicates; zinc and iron phytates associated with calcium)

Table 2 (contd.)

Chemical speciation of ETE in the diet

a) *Synergisms enhancing mobility of element*:

   enhancing absorption (e.g., citrate, histidine, enhancing zinc absorption; ascorbate modifying iron/copper antagonism)

   maintaining systemic transport and mobility of some elements (e.g., transferrins, albumins and other plasma ligands)

b) *Antagonisms limiting mobility of element*:

   decreasing gastrointestinal lumen solubility of elements (e.g., calcium/zinc/phytate, copper/sulfides)

   competing with element for receptors involved in absorption, transport, storage or function (e.g., cadmium/zinc/copper antagonism)

   mechanisms unknown (e.g., iron/copper, iron/zinc antagonism)

Fetal requirements for ETEs result in increased maternal requirements, as discussed in section 4.5.

4.3.2 Infancy

The gastrointestinal tract, liver and kidneys of the newborn are functionally immature and may not have the ability to achieve homeostatic regulation of the uptake of ETEs or to discriminate against toxic metals (Mills, 1985; WHO, 1996). Much of what is known about gastrointestinal absorption during infancy is derived from animal studies. Few studies have been conducted on humans (WHO, 1996). Brain development is affected by post-natal deficiencies in iodine (Bleichrodt & Born, 1994).

4.3.3 The elderly

The efficiency of intestinal uptake of some trace elements declines in the elderly (Bunker et al., 1984). On a diet of 15 mg zinc/day, men aged 65 to 74 years absorbed 17% of dietary zinc, in contrast to 33%

absorbed by 22- to 33-year-old males (Turnlund et al., 1986). Absorption of chromium and selenium does not appear to be significantly different for elderly subjects (Anderson & Kozlowsky, 1985).

4.4 Variability due to gender

Gender differences in nutritional requirements are a consequence of various metabolic differences between the two sexes. For example, women have only about two-thirds the fat-free body mass (FFM) of men, while having a larger percentage of body fat. The male-female ratio for urinary creatinine excretion (an index of muscle mass) is 1.5. Males are also generally larger in stature than females. Skeletal size is a function of height as is body calcium. Because adult females have only two-thirds as much FFM as males, protein and energy requirements are correspondingly less. Basal metabolic rate is more closely related to FFM than it is to total body weight, so that total energy requirements are less for women than men (Forbes, 1996). These differences have an impact on body content of minerals including ETEs. Other significant gender differences include iron losses during menstruation and loss of zinc in seminal fluid (Yip & Dallman, 1996; WHO, 1996). Differences in requirements for specific ETEs are noted in the examples cited in section 6.

4.5 Pregnancy and lactation

Pregnancy and lactation increase demand for some ETEs, particularly copper, zinc, iron and iodine (Picciano, 1996).

The increased dietary recommendation for copper in pregnancy is about 100 µg per day (IOM, 2001). During lactation, the amount of copper secreted in the milk is about 200 µg per day, which increases the dietary requirement for copper (WHO, 1996; IOM 2001).

Pregnancy increases the dietary requirement for zinc by about 3 mg/day (IOM, 2001). An increase in intestinal absorption during pregnancy partially offsets the increased needs of the developing fetus and neonate. Lactating women need an additional 4–7 mg zinc per day (Yang & Chen, 1993; IOM, 2001).

Additional iron is required to support the growth of the placenta, transfer to the fetus, increase in red blood cell mass and loss during delivery. In some women, this extra need may be accommodated by sufficient iron stores, lack of menstrual losses and homeostatic adaptation, provided the dietary intake is adequate. However, many women require iron supplements during pregnancy (BNF, 1995).

Maternal iodine deficiency may produce fetal hypothyroidism resulting in cretinism (Hetzel, 1989; Stanbury, 1996). Recommended iodine intake during pregnancy is 200 µg/day (WHO, 1996). In China, over 400 million people live in iodine deficiency endemic areas (National Iodine Deficiency Disorder (IDD) Surveillance Group, 2000; Chen, 2000). Over 1.5 billion people worldwide have iodine intakes close to one-half this amount and are at risk of developing iodine-deficiency disorders (WHO, 1996).

4.6 Chemical species of ETEs

The chemical species of an ETE that is ingested may influence its solubility and bioavailability for gastrointestinal absorption, and, in many instances, alter the risks of deficiency and excess. These are important considerations in the risk assessment of an ETE. For example, in aqueous solutions iron exists in two oxidation states: Fe(II), the ferrous form, and Fe(III), the ferric form. The ferrous form is better absorbed than the ferric form, although reduction of ferric to ferrous iron readily occurs in the gastrointestinal tract at acidic pH (WHO, 1996). Iron salts in dairy products and vegetables account for approximately 40% of the diet in women in the USA, 31% coming from meat sources and 25% from food fortification (mainly cereal and wheat-based products) (Yip & Dallman, 1996). Iron in foods of vegetable origin is less well absorbed than haem iron in meat. Ascorbic acid enhances iron absorption; calcium, phosphates and phytates in cereals tend to inhibit absorption (Yip & Dallman, 1996). Chemical speciation and solubility affect copper absorption. $CuSO_4$ is easily absorbed, CuO is less well absorbed and insoluble compounds such as CuS are essentially not absorbed (IPCS, 1998). Water-soluble forms of selenium are efficiently absorbed (80–90%), while absorption of elemental selenium and selenium sulfide is lower (Robinson, 1989; Butler et al., 1991). The systemic metabolism of organic and inorganic forms of selenium differs and this will affect the efficiency of conversion into biologically active forms, as well as the toxicity of the element, e.g., seleno-methionine is non-specifically incorporated into plasma and body proteins, while inorganic selenium forms have less effect on tissue concentrations (Butler et al., 1991).

4.7 Interactions between ETEs

Interactions amongst ETEs must be considered in their risk assessment. For example, important interactions may occur during absorption and metabolism. Interactions between ETEs are summarized in WHO (1996) and IPCS (1998, 2001). The following examples indicate that information regarding factors that influence absorption and bioavailability exists. A more data-related approach for assessing toxicological risk for nutritionally essential trace elements may be possible, particularly if relevant information has been previously used to determine RDAs. Such interactions become crucial in the interpretation of results of experimental studies and their relevance to human health. The interactions described are dependent on dose, source and nature of diet, and previous nutritional status. The examples provided are just examples and by no means provide a comprehensive account.

4.7.1 Copper and zinc

Copper has the potential for a variety of interactions with other nutrients, particularly other ETEs, which may be regulated, in part or fully, by the processes of gastrointestinal absorption. The relationship with zinc is perhaps the best characterized. High zinc intakes (50 mg or more per day) inhibit absorption of copper by competing directly for serosal transport in the gut or by inducing metallothionein in the intestinal cells. Zinc is a good inducer of metallothionein but copper has a higher affinity for the protein. Zinc and copper may co-exist on metallothionein and the zinc-induced metallothionein may sequester the copper and retard its transport across the serosal membrane. Consequences of the high affinity of copper for zinc-induced metallothionein can be both negative (i.e. excessive ingestion of zinc may promote copper deficiency) or positive (i.e. use of high zinc level as a therapeutic agent in the treatment of Wilson's disease) (IPCS, 1998). Copper and, to a lesser extent, zinc are mobilized from renal metallothionein during pregnancy. The amount of copper bound to metallothionein in the kidney during pregnancy decreases whereas that of zinc increases. Zinc may be more available during pregnancy than tissue copper (Suzuki et al., 1990).

4.7.2 Selenium and iodine

The metabolism of selenium and iodine is interrelated in the conversion of thyroxine to triiodothyronine (T_4 to T_3) by selenium-containing deiodinase enzymes. Triiodothyronine is crucial for brain development in the fetus. The triiodothyronine must be formed from thyroxine in the cells of the brain by the enzyme type II iodothyronine deiodinase, a selenoprotein (Davey et al., 1995), because it does not have free access to the brain from serum. Animal studies have shown that combined selenium and iodine deficiencies leads to more severe hypothyroidism than does iodine deficiency alone, and there is some evidence that cretinism in newborn babies may be the result of combined deficiencies of selenium and iodine (Arthur & Beckett, 1994). While the implications in humans are as yet uncertain, one study suggests that effects of iodine deficiency are worsened if selenium status is low (WHO, 1996). Selenium supplementation in iodine deficient areas may aggravate the effects of iodine deficiency on fetal brain development (Frey, 1995).

4.8 Genetically determined human variability and disorders of homeostasis

There are a number of disorders in homeostatic mechanisms that can result in deficiency or excess from exposure to ETE at levels that are within the AROI for the general population (IPCS, 1998). Wilson's disease (prevalence of 1 in 30 000) and Menkes disease (prevalence of 1 in 200 000) are heredity disorders of copper metabolism. In Wilson's disease the fundamental defect is believed to be impaired biliary excretion of copper resulting in copper accumulation in most organs of the body, particularly the liver, brain and kidney, which provide the most apparent clinical manifestations. This subpopulation develops disease in the deficiency range of the AROI for the general population.

Menkes disease is an X-linked recessive disorder of copper metabolism that resembles a copper deficiency state regardless of the level of copper intake above the AROI for the general population. It results from a defect in the gene coding for a P-type transporting ATPase, resulting in a marked reduction in the first phase of copper transport (IPCS, 1998).

Indian childhood cirrhosis (ICC) is an insidious disease of the liver progressing to cirrhosis. It is characterized by increases in copper levels in serum and liver. The etiology is uncertain but in some studies (but not all) it seems to be related to relative excess copper exposure from boiling and storing milk in copper-yielding brass containers (IPCS, 1998). However, the disorder sometimes occurs in multiple family members, suggesting a genetic component. Similar disorders have been described in other countries and referred to as idiopathic copper toxicosis or non-Indian childhood cirrhosis. On the basis of pedigree analysis, the cause seems to be an autosomal recessive condition leading to increased sensitivity to high copper intake (Müller et al., 1998).

In Caucasian populations, haemochromatosis is a very common inherited disorder in iron homeostasis (Crawford et al., 1996). The specific genetic defect has been identified (Feder et al., 1996). The disease is characterized by excessive iron absorption, elevated plasma iron concentration, transferrin saturation, and altered distribution of iron stores. The liver is the organ with the greatest concentration of iron, and mixed macromicronodular cirrhosis can eventually occur in cases of heavy iron loading. Data from Canada suggest the prevalence of this disorder may be ~0.3% for homozygotes and > 11% for heterozygotes; the risks associated with heterozygotes need to be established (Borwein et al., 1983).

4.9 Acquired disorders of homeostasis

There are several acquired pathological states that might result in elevated requirements for ETEs. These are very important issues and need to be given special considerations that go beyond the framework of a risk assessment of an ETE for the general population. Examples include patients with clinical malabsorption syndromes, excessive gastrointestinal losses of ETEs, catabolic states or patients on total parental nutrition.

5. EFFECTS OF DEFICIENCY AND EXCESS

5.1 Range in severity of effects

Health effects from deficiency or excess may range from lethal effects through clinical effects to subclinical effects, with or without functional significance, as shown in Fig. 5. While lethal effects and clinical disease must always be prevented, subclinical effects indicating impairment of organ function are often identified as critical effects. A number of biochemical changes such as enzyme activities are often used as biomarkers to assess various levels of intake of ETEs. Biochemical effects without functional significance (curves 4 and 5 in Fig. 5) are considered without health impact and should not be regarded as critical effects.

A number of examples are provided below for different levels of severity. It should be recognized, however, that spectrum of effects may be a continuum influenced not only by dose, but also reversibility, timing and duration of exposure and interactions, as well as by other factors that influence variability in response as reviewed in section 4.

It should be noted, however, that there is no assumption that the shapes of the curves for deficiency and toxicity are necessarily symmetrical or similar in slope. In addition, the assessment of severity must consider the number of individuals affected.

5.2 Comparability of end-points used to define deficiency and excess

There is a broad range in the severity of effects from deficiency of ETEs and toxicity as shown in Fig. 5. The severity of health effects to be applied in assessing risks from deficiency or toxicity from exposure to ETEs should be comparable. Fig. 5 shows a set of theoretical curves in order to illustrate the results of application of criteria that would result in similar severity of end-points in populations from deficiency and excess. Although markers of marginal deficiency states and minimal or subclinical toxicity are often lacking, it is the objective of this monograph to provide both toxicologists and nutritionists with the methodologies to determine boundaries of the AROI that have been

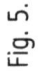

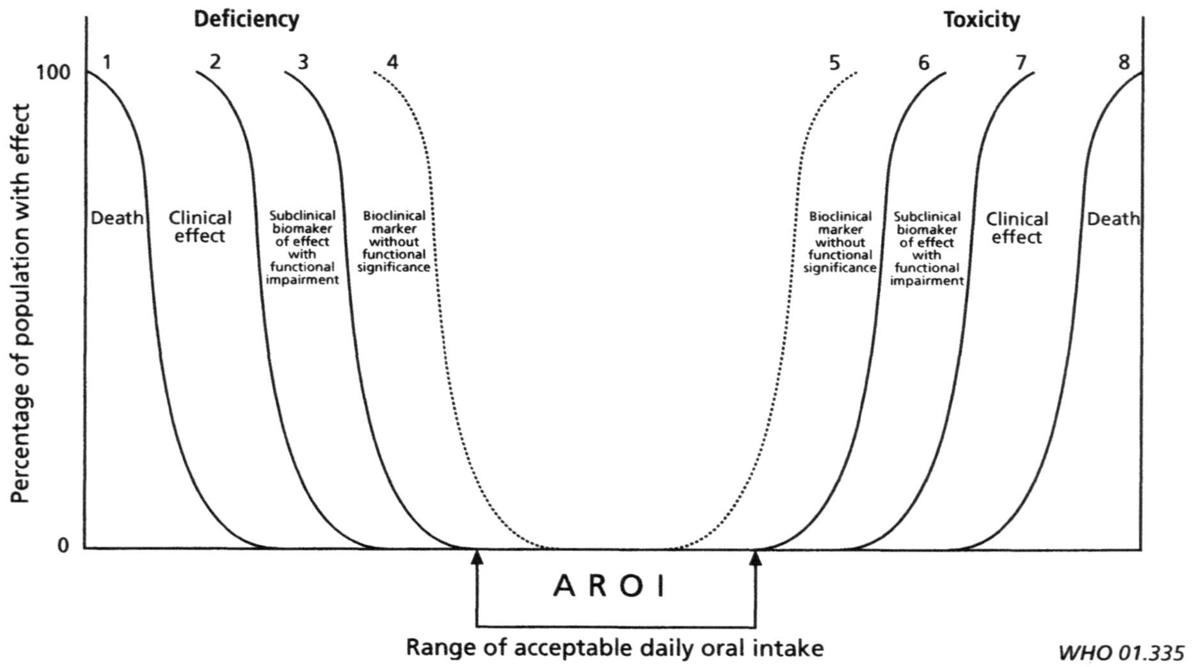

Fig. 5. Theoretical dose-response curves for various effects occurring in a population at various levels of intake (doses) of an ETE.

The lower end of the dose response curve for such critical effects related to deficiency (curve 3) and toxicity (curve 6) defines the range of acceptable daily oral intakes.

defined by end-points of comparable significance. The following examples illustrate the range of end-points encountered.

5.2.1 Range of clinical and biochemical markers of deficiency and excess

Exposures to deficient or excessive amounts of ETEs induce a range of clinical and biochemical end-points. This range off effects extends from lethality to subclinical and biochemical changes, which include evidence of homeostasis.

5.2.1.1 Deficiency

Lethal dietary deficiency can occur as the result of extreme deficiency of a single ETE. However, lethal outcomes more often occur as the consequence of nutritional starvation and deficiencies of multiple ETEs, sometimes in association with infection or increased susceptibility, as in a sensitive subgroup population. For most ETEs clinical conditions associated with deficiency have been well described (Fe, Cu, Zn, Se) (WHO, 1996; Yip & Dallman, 1996).

A number of subclinical biomarkers, such as changes in levels of enzyme activity, have been shown to occur in people with low intakes of some ETEs. In some cases the change in enzyme level is of functional significance and may even be the precursor of clinical disease. In other cases, decreases may not be associated with any demonstrable functional effect. The relationship to functional change may reflect whether the enzyme level is normally well above that which is rate-limiting in the pathway so that small quantitative changes are not reflected in a functional change.

Criteria for determining when such changes are physiological adaptations or adverse health effects have not been established. As in all toxicological assessments, the critical effect or health end-point must be determined. The main difficulty is establishing whether an effect is to be considered biologically significant or non-significant.

5.2.1.2 Excess

Death and disease related to acute or chronic exposure/intake have been documented for some of the ETEs (Mertz, 1987; WHO, 1996).

Clinical effects by definition include objective signs and/or subject-perceived symptoms, but they may not be specific to particular excessive exposure. In some situations the biological effect of excess may be due to other intervening factors, as noted in sections 4, such as genetic predisposition or acquired pathological states. In these cases it is particularly difficult to establish a causal relationship unless controlled studies are available. There are few instances where this type of information is available for ETEs.

Subclinical effects encompass laboratory measures of different types (biochemical, physiological, immunological, metabolic balances). Subclinical indices may serve to indicate risk of future clinical disease. The strength of the relationship between subclinical effects and disease or risk of disease is crucial to the evaluation of the significance of the effect. Similar to the situation with biochemical markers of deficiency, subclinical markers of toxicity have been identified from exposure to ETEs. In order to use a biomarker as a critical effect, one must determine whether it signals a subclinical stage of disease or abnormality of organ function. Unfortunately, for several potentially useful markers there is a lack of such information and further definition of the clinical and functional significance of biomarkers is needed.

5.2.2 Examples of range of effects

5.2.2.1 Iron

Severe iron deficiency may lead to severe anaemia with lethal outcome in rare cases (Kushner, 1985). Anaemia, as it occurs in iron deficiency in young children and sometimes in women of child-bearing age, will produce clinically apparent pallor, fatigue and susceptibility to infections. In addition, psychomotor development has been shown to be impaired in children with iron-deficiency anaemia (Walter et al., 1989).

When iron intake is low, serum ferritin levels decrease or fall as stores are depleted. Serum transferrin receptor levels increase as tissue requirement for iron increase and there is decreased transferrin saturation and increased erythrocyte protoporphyrin. While these markers are excellent indicators of low body iron stores, the clinical significance of change in a single marker is unclear and it may be

Effects of Deficiency and Excess

necessary to look at a battery of biomarkers to interpret clinical significance (Yip & Dallman, 1996; WHO, 2001). Low serum ferritin concentration in young women without anaemia is associated with a reduction of maximal oxygen consumption, as demonstrated in physical performance tests (Zhu & Haas, 1997), and an increase in adverse pregnancy outcomes (Scholl & Hediger, 1994; BNF, 1995).

Increased levels of serum ferritin and transferrin are indicators of excessive iron intake and iron overload (Borch-Iohnsen et al., 1995). Ingestion of excessive amounts of soluble iron salts gives rise to gastrointestinal manifestations with vomiting and diarrhoea, often with bloody stools, and chronic high exposures may lead to liver cirrhosis (Borch-Iohnsen et al., 1995). The clinical effects from iron overload are increased risks of cardiomyopathy and hepatic cancer (Bradbear et al., 1985; Niederau et al., 1985). It is possible that systemic iron overload might also predispose to cancer in other organs, but the evidence for this, such as that based on surveys of patients with genetic haemochromatosis is not conclusive. It has also been suggested that patients with high serum ferritin level as evidence of exposure to iron are at a increased risk of colonic adenoma and possibly colonic cancer. However, a clearly causal association between oral intake of iron and any risk of cancer of the colon or any other organs has not been shown (Stevens, 1996). Some studies have proposed a link between high iron intake and coronary heart disease (Tuomainen et al., 1998; Klipstein-Grobusch et al., 1999), but a meta-analysis of prospective studies did not support this relationship (Danesh & Appleby, 1999).

5.2.2.2 Zinc

In deriving the AROI for zinc there are difficulties in identifying appropriate end-points (WHO 1996). Zinc deficiency produces growth failures, poor immunity, impaired wound healing and impairment of special senses and cognition (Sandstead, 1993; IPCS, 1998). While there are many sensitive biomarkers, none are specific to zinc. Monitoring target enzymes during controlled repletion studies may be the most specific test of dietary deficiency (O'Donnell, 1997). The estimates of requirements may be evaluated by factorial estimates, i.e. by adding together the requirements for tissue growth, maintenance, metabolism and endogenous losses, and adjusting for increased efficiency of absorption (WHO, 1996; IOM, 2001).

Homeostatic mechanisms maintain plasma and tissue zinc concentrations over a long period of time at low intakes by increased absorption and reduction in losses of endogenous zinc (WHO, 1996; IPCS, 2001). When intakes are at the basal requirement level (Fig. 4), the ability to increase the efficiency of zinc retention has been fully exploited. For adult males an uptake of 1.4 mg/day has been judged to maintain zinc equilibrium without the need of adaptive changes in endogenous losses. With 30% fractional uptake from the diet, this corresponds to a normative dietary requirement of 4.7 mg/day. Lacking corresponding long-term studies in other age groups, endogenous losses in relation to basal metabolic rates for adults have been used as the basis for extrapolation (WHO, 1996).

There are a number of biomarkers for zinc excess including decreased erythrocyte superoxide dismutase (E-SOD) activity and decreased cytochrome c oxidase activity in platelets, and reduced serum ferritin concentrations, caused by the effects of zinc on copper and iron, respectively. None of these are specific or reliable indicators of excess exposure in an individual, but they may assist in considering population exposure (O'Donnell, 1997).

5.2.2.3 Copper

Severe copper deficiency can result in defective connective tissue synthesis and oesteogenesis, nutropena and iron-resistant anaemia (WHO, 1996). Low copper intake results in decreases in ceruloplasmin levels and superoxide dismutase (SOD) (IPCS, 1998). Single acute or repeated ingestion of large doses of copper may induce gastrointestinal toxicity. This may be followed by haematuria, jaundice and multiple organ failure and death. Chronic exposure to high doses of copper can lead to liver damage (IPCS, 1998).

5.2.2.4 Selenium

In China, Keshan disease, which is a result of selenium deficiency, possibly in combination with infection, may produce myocardial abnormalities and sometimes death (Chen et al., 1980). Supplementation and improved nutrition has been shown to prevent this condition (Keshan Disease Research Group of the Chinese Academy of Medical Science, 1979; Lin, 1989; Alexander, 1993; Zhang, 1998).

Effects of Deficiency and Excess

Selenocysteine is the active component of oxidases such as glutathione peroxidases and deiodinases. The effects of low selenium intake on deiodinases may cause changes in thyroid hormone function. Selenium deficiency also results in incomplete saturation of glutathione peroxidase (GSHPx) in plasma, erythrocytes and platelets. The clinical or health significance of incomplete GSHPx saturation is uncertain particularly in the most sensitive compartment, i.e. platelets. Incomplete GSHPx saturation in plasma does not occur until selenium intake falls below approximately 40 µg/day (Yang et al., 1989a,b). WHO (1996) used the intake necessary to obtain two-thirds of maximum plasma glutathione peroxidase activity as the criterion for normative requirement.

Ingestion of high doses of selenium salts causes nausea, vomiting and subsequent neurological disease, hair and nail changes and skin lesions. Chronic high-dose exposure may give rise to a range of clinical expressions, such as neurological, skin, nail and hair changes and also liver dysfunction manifested by a prolonged prothrombin time and increases in alanine aminotransferase activity (Alexander et al., 1988; Alexander & Meltzer, 1995).

Clinical signs of selenosis are observed at and above intakes of 900 µg/day (WHO, 1996). Biochemical effects in the form of a reduction of the ratio of selenium in plasma to that in erythrocytes were seen at daily intakes of 750–800 µg (Yang et al., 1989). A maximal daily safe dietary selenium intake of 400 µg has been suggested for adults (WHO, 1996). This figure was derived arbitrarily by dividing the mean marginal level of daily safe dietary selenium intake, defined as 800 µg, by an uncertainty factor of 2.

6. APPLICATION OF HOMEOSTATIC MODEL IN HUMAN HEALTH RISK ASSESSMENT TO EXPOSURE TO ETEs

6.1 Summary of principles

Principles underlying the use of the "homeostatic model" are summarized in Table 3. Many of these principles were examined at a workshop in 1992 (Mertz, 1993; Mertz et al., 1994) and have been discussed in general in previous sections of this monograph. Application of these principles should provide guidance on the acceptable oral exposure range for any ETE.

In using the homeostatic model, an important consideration is physiological adaptation to changing levels of ingestion. This adaptation is applicable to risk assessment for ETEs. Sources of variation when estimating acceptable ranges of oral intakes include person-based variables (e.g., age, gender, physiological status) and variation in efficiency of absorption from the food and water that provide these elements. This approach of setting acceptable ranges (AROI) in the presence of physiological adaptation to changing levels of ingestion is applicable to risk assessment for ETEs only and is not meant to apply to trace elements that are not recognized as essential for humans.

The lower and upper limits of physiological adaptation differ for individual elements. For example, the anions fluoride and iodide are readily absorbed and changes in excretion rates are the main determinant of quantities retained. Some cations (e.g., iron) are predominantly maintained by control of absorption at the intestinal level. However, copper and zinc are controlled by both absorption and excretion. Data identifying the levels of intake that exceed the capacity of homeostatic mechanisms are typically not available, and additional research on this topic is recommended to reduce reliance on default values.

Fractional absorption of trace elements and the capacity for physiological adaptation varies with age, gender and physiological

Table 3 Principles underlying use of the homeostatic model in
human health risk assessment of ETEs

- Homeostatic mechanisms should be identified for the selected ETE.

- Variations of the population's homeostatic adaptation must be considered.

- There is a "zone of safe and adequate exposure for each defined age and gender groups" for all ETEs – a zone compatible with good health. This is the acceptable range of oral intake (AROI).

- All appropriate scientific disciplines must be involved in developing an AROI.

- Data on toxicity and deficiency should receive equal critical evaluation.

- Bioavailability should be considered in assessing the effects of deficiency and toxicity.

- Nutrient interactions should be considered when known.

- Chemical species and the route and duration of exposure should be fully described.

- Biological end-points used to define the lower (RDA) and upper (toxic) boundaries of the AROI should ideally have similar degrees of functional significance. This is particularly relevant where there is a potentially narrow AROI as a result of one end-point being of negligible clinical significance.

- All appropriate data should be used to determine the dose–response curve for establishing the boundaries of the AROI.

status (e.g., pregnancy, lactation), as well as systemic need and burden of the ETE. Likewise, nutritional requirements and levels associated with toxicity and deficiency differ with individual variables. Ultimately the goal is to produce a range of intakes that meet nutritional requirements and identify intakes associated with toxicity for specific age-gender groupings that do not overlap. However, when comparisons are made for a range of age-gender groups, the derived deficit and toxicity curves may overlap. Careful interpretation of estimates of acceptable ranges of oral intakes for multiple age-gender specific populations is necessary to establish tolerable concentrations of an element in food and/or water, as well as in soil when appropriate.

Variability occurs despite homeostatic adaptation, which, over time, smoothes out and regulates the body burden and compensates for variability in intake and bioavailability. There is variability in some of the factors cited in Table 3, which is independent of nutritional factors and which will need to be appreciated if these factors are to be used to set the AROI. The traditional use of UF/SF will increase the likelihood of overlap.

Conceptually, another important factor in setting the AROI is the variability in the measurement selected as a marker of an adverse effect.

6.2 Scheme for application of principles

Fig. 6 depicts the steps that should be followed in applying the "homeostatic model" for assessment of health risk from exposure to ETEs. In reading the steps summarized in Fig. 6, it is essential that the detailed description of the principles and the scientific support for these principles, found elsewhere in the text of this monograph or in the references cited, be consulted. In all steps it is essential that uncertainty and variability in the database and population of concern be identified. Application of the principles requires a multidisciplinary scientific assessment, using data on both deficiency and excess exposures.

Application of Homeostatic Model

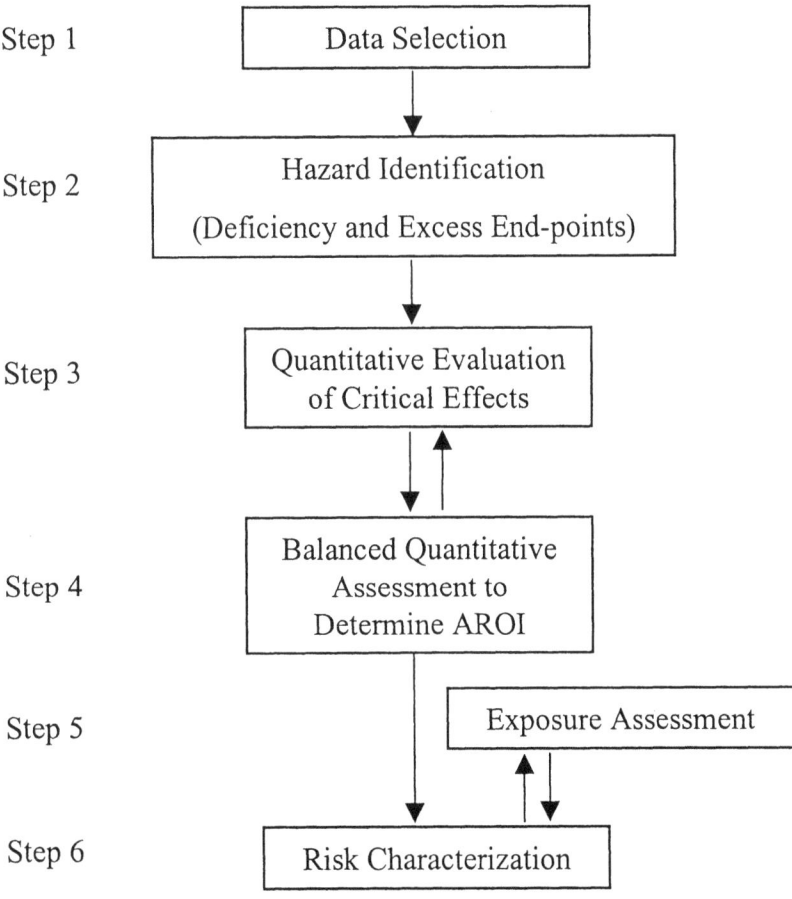

Fig. 6. Application of the principles for the assessment of risk from essential trace elements

Step 1 The first step is to collect relevant data on the ETE and evaluate its adequacy. The objective of this step is to develop a database for further analyses. When there are insufficient human data to evaluate a functional effect, then it may be useful to have supportive animal data.

Step 2 A weight of evidence approach must be used to identify clinically and toxicologically relevant end-points from deficiency as well as from excess exposure. Amongst the factors considered in establishing these end-points are chemical species, homeostatic mechanisms, bioavailability, nature of exposure, population variability and age-sex variation (see Chapter 4). A practical definition for biological significance is the capacity of the biological indicator to predict the occurrence of deficiency or toxicity. While some examples are provided in Chapter 5, most biochemical or functional biomarkers have not been validated in terms of their ability to anticipate the occurrence of adverse effects. The successful application of this step requires the cooperative expertise of all appropriate scientific disciplines.

Step 3 Various dose–response curves for each end-point from deficient and excess exposure in various populations need to be described and evaluated. Levels of exposures/intakes that are responsible for the occurrence of critical effects may be derived from case reports and experimental, epidemiological, clinical or metabolic studies by both nutritionists and toxicologists.

Step 4 AROIs are derived using a balanced approach weighing the effects seen after both deficient and excess exposures in healthy populations. In deriving the AROI, the most sensitive validated biomarkers of subclinical and toxicological effects should be used. Methodology for determining the levels to prevent deficient and excess exposure in the population subgroups is described in Chapter 3. The health significance of these effects should be as comparable as possible. There are difficulties in establishing end-points of comparable health significance. When human data are inadequate, animal studies may be used to help establish the upper or lower limits of AROI.

Step 5 Exposure assessment identifies and quantifies exposure sources (e.g., water, food, supplements, and soil and dust), bioavailability and exposure patterns for subgroups of the population (IPCS, 2000). This will include the relevant timing and duration of exposures for the relevant health end-points. There should be assessment of the variability of the magnitude of intake (e.g., by using intake percentiles for the relevant population) and the source of intake (e.g., the changing fractions between food and water). There should also be assessments of subpopulations that have distinct patterns of consumption, perhaps for social or cultural reasons (US EPA, 1992). Age-associated differences in caloric and fluid intake should also be considered (ILSI, 1992).

Step 6 Risk characterization iteratively integrates the available exposure information and the AROI. This process takes into consideration the variability, exposure and dose–response for multiple subpopulations, evaluating the strengths and weaknesses of each step (IPCS, 1999). The risk characterization should be validated by a variety of means. Risk characterization must be transparent, so that the conclusions drawn from scientific assessment are identified separately from policy judgements, and the use of default values or methods and of assumptions in the risk assessment are clearly identified (Younes et al., 1998). It also requires the identification of the subgroup of greatest concern from nutritional and toxicological perspectives. Once an AROI is in place, there should be a mechanism for reviewing new data and, if necessary, updating the AROI. Research needs should be identified to fill gaps in the data.

7. RECOMMENDATIONS

It is recommended that:

- the principles for development of AROIs in risk assessment of ETEs elaborated in this monograph be followed in all future consideration of ETEs; these principles may be applied to any nutrient;

- updating of this monograph continues appropriately;

- all relevant disciplines be involved in future developments;

- this monograph be used as a contribution to the ongoing process of harmonization of approaches to risk assessment;

- encouragement be given to the acquisition, development and interpretation of exposure data for ETEs for population groups;

- greater emphasis be given to risk characterization, emphasizing the strengths and weaknesses of the hazard identification, dose–response and exposure assessment components in order to increase the transparency of the process;

- the terminology used in determining and applying the AROI be harmonized.

8. FURTHER RESEARCH

It is recommended that:

- priority be given to the support of those areas where critical data are lacking for the derivation of AROIs for ETEs;

- specific and sensitive biomarkers representative of homeostatic mechanisms at the boundaries of deficient and excess exposure to ETEs be identified and validated;

- support be given to the use of biomarkers in the development of dose–response curves embracing customary dietary intakes;

- support be given to systematic and integrated evaluation and use of biomarkers for the development of AROIs in populations of interest.

REFERENCES

Abernathy CO, Cantilli R, Du JT, & Levander OA (1993) Essentiality versus toxicity: some considerations in the risk assessment of essential elements. In: Saxena J, ed. Hazard assessment of chemicals. Washington, DC, Taylor & Francis, pp 81-113.

Alexander J (1993) Risk assessment of selenium. Scand J Work Environ Health, **19**: 122-123.

Alexander J & Meltzer HM (1995) Selenium. In Oskarsson A. ed Risk evaluation of essential trace elements - Essential versus toxic levels of intake. Copenhagen, Nordic Council of Ministers, pp 15-65.

Alexander J, Hogberg J, Thomassen Y, & Asseth J (1988) Selenium. In: Seiler HG & Sigel H eds. Handbook of toxicity of inorganic compounds. New York, Marcel Dekker, Inc., pp 581-588.

Allen LH (1997) Pregnancy and iron deficiency: Unresolved issues. Nutr Rev, **55**: 91-101.

Anderson GJ (1996) Control of iron absorption. J Gastroenterol Hepatol, **11**: 1030-1032.

Anderson RH & Kozlowsky AS (1985) Chromium intake, absorption and excretion of subjects consuming self-selected diets. Am J Clin Nutr, **41**: 1177-1183.

Andrews NC (1999) The iron transporter DMT1. Int J Biochem Cell Biol, **31**: 991-994.

Arthur JR & Beckett GJ (1994) Roles of selenium in type I iodothyronine 5'-deiodinase and in thyroid hormone and iodine metabolism. In: Burk RF, ed. Selenium in biology and human health. New York, Springer-Verlag, pp 93-115.

Baer M & King J (1984) Tissue zinc levels and zinc excretion during experimental zinc depletion in young men. Am J Clin Nutr, **39**: 556-570.

Barclay SM, Aggett PJ, Lloyd DJ, & Duffty P (1991) Reduced erythrocyte superoxide dismutase activity in low birth weight infants given iron supplements. Pediatr Res, **29**: 297-301.

Beck BD, Rudel R, Hook GC, & Bowers TS (1995) Risk Assessment. In: Goyer RA, Klaassen CD, Waalkes MP, eds. Metal toxicology. San Diego, Academic Press, pp 141-186.

Becking GC (1997) Risk assessment for essential trace elements: a homeostatic model. In: Langley A, Mangas S, eds. Zinc: report of an international meeting, September 1996, Adelaide, SA. Adelaide, South Australian Health Commission, National Environmental Health Forum Monographs, Metal series No. 2, pp 16-30.

Black MR, Mederios DM, Burnett E, & Welke R (1988) Zinc supplements and serum lipids in adult white males. Am J Clin Nutr, **47**: 970-975.

Bleichrodt N & Born MP (1994) A meta-analysis of research on iodine and its relationship to cognitive development. In: Stanbury JB ed. The damaged brain of iodine deficiency. Cognitive behavioral, neuromotor, and educative aspects. New York. Cognizant Communication, pp 195-200.

References

Bloomfield J, Dixon SR, & McCredie DA (1971) Potential hepatotoxicity of copper in recurrent hemodialysis. Arch Int Med, **128**: 555-560.

BNF (1995) Iron: Nutritional and physiological significance. Report of the British Nutrition Foundation Task Force. London, Chapman & Hall, pp 110-123.

Bodwell CE & Erdan JW Jr eds. (1988) Nutrient interactions. Institute of Food Technologists (IFT) Basic Symposium Series. New York, Marcel Dekker, 379 pp.

Borch-Iohnsen B & Petersson-Grawe K (1995) Iron. In: Oskarsson A ed. Risk evaluation of essential trace elements - essential versus toxic levels of intake. Copenhagen, Nordic Council of Ministers, pp 67-118.

Borwein ST, Ghent CN, Flanagan PR, Chamberlain MJ, & Valberg LS (1983) Genetic and phenotypic expression of hemochromatosis in Canadians. Clin Invest Med, **6**: 171-179.

Bowman BA & Risher JF (1994) Comparison of the methodology approaches used in the derivation of recommended dietary allowances and oral reference doses for nutritionally essential elements. In: Mertz W, Abernathy CO, & Olin SS eds. Risk assessment of essential elements. Washington, DC, ILSI Press, pp 63-76.

Bradbear RA, Bain C, & Siskind V (1985) Cohort study of internal malignancy in genetic hemochromatosis and other chronic non-alcoholic liver diseases. J Natl Cancer Inst, **75**: 81-85.

Bremner I & Beattie JH (1995) Copper and zinc metabolism in health and disease: speciation and interactions. Proc Nutr Soc, **54**: 489-499.

Brewer GJ, Johnson V, Dick RD, Kluin KJ, Fink JK, & Brunberg JA (1996) Treatment of Wilson disease with ammonium tetrathimolybdate. II. Initial therapy in 33 neurologically affected patients and follow-up with zinc therapy. Arch Neurol, **53**: 1017-1025.

Bunker VW, Hinks LJ, Lawson MS, & Clayton BE (1984) Assessment of zinc and copper status of elderly people using metabolic balance studies and measurements of leucocyte concentrations. Am J Clin Nutr, **40**: 1096-1102.

Butler JA, Thomson CD, Whanger PD, & Robinson MF (1991) Selenium distribution in blood fractions of New Zealand women taking organic or inorganic selenium. Am J Clin Nutr, **53**: 748-754.

Camakaris J, Voskoboinik I, & Mercer JF (1999) Molecular mechanisms of copper homeostasis. Biochem Biophys Res Commun, **261**: 225-232.

Cantilli R, Abernathy CO, & Donohue JM (1994) Derivation of the reference dose for zinc. In: Mertz W, Abernathy CO, & Olin SS eds. Risk assessment of essential elements. Washington, DC, ILSI Press, pp 113-125.

Chandra RK (1984) Excessive intake of zinc impairs immune responses. JAMA, **252**: 1443-1446.

Chen ZB (2000) [Current status and perspectives on prevention and treatment of Iodine deficiency disorders (IDD) in China.] Chinese J Epidemiology, **19**: 1-2 (in Chinese).

Chen X, Yang G, Chen J, Wen Z, & Gen K (1980) Studies on the relations of selenium and Keshan disease. Biol Trace Elem Res, **2**: 91-107.

Christie GL & Williams DR (1995) Classification of metal ions in living systems. In: Berthon G ed. Handbook of metal-ligand interactions in biological fluids. Volume 1. Bioinorganic medicine. New York, Marcel Dekker, Inc, pp 29-37.

Conrad ME (1993) Regulation of iron absorption. Prog Clin Biol Res, **380**: 203-219.

Cousins RJ (1985) Absorption, transport, and hepatic metabolism of copper and zinc: special reference to metallothionein and ceruloplasmin. Physiol Rev, **65**: 238-259.

Cousins RJ (1996) Zinc. In: Ziegler EE & Filer LJ eds. Recent knowledge in nutrition. Washington, DC, ILSI Press, pp 293-306.

Cousins RJ & McMahon RJ (2000) Integrative aspects of zinc transporters. J Nutr, **130**: 1384-1387.

Cox DW (1999) Disorders of copper transport. Br Med Bull, **55**: 544-555.

Crawford DHG, Powell LW, & Halliday JW (1996) Factors influencing disease expression in hemochromatosis. Ann Rev Nutr, **16**: 139-160.

Crump KS (1984) A new method for determining allowable daily intakes. Fundam Appl Toxicol, **4**: 854-871.

Cunningham J, Fu A, Mearkle PL, & Brown RL (1994) Hyperzincuria in individuals with insulin-dependent diabetes mellitus: concurrent zinc status and the effect of high-dose zinc supplementation. Metabol, **43**: 1558-1562.

Davey JC, Becker KB, Schneider MJ, St Germain DL, & Galton VA (1995) Cloning of a cDNA for the type II iodothyronine deiodinase. J Biol Chem, **270**: 26786-26789.

Danesh J & Appleby P (1999) Coronary heart disease and iron status: Meta-analyses of prospective studies. Circulation, **99**: 852-854.

Donaldson RM & Barreras RF (1965) Intestinal absorption of trace quantities of chromium. J Lab Clin Med, **68**: 484-493.

Donovan A, Brownlie A, Zhou Y, Shepard J, Pratt S, Moynihan J, Paw BH, Drejer A, Barut B, Zapata A, Law TC, Brugnara C, Lux SE, Pinkus GS, Pinkus JL, Kingsley PD, Palls J, Fleming MD, Andrews NC, Zon LI (2000) Positional cloning of zebrafish ferroportin 1 identifies a conserved vertebrate iron exporter. Nature, **403**: 776-781.

Dourson M (1994) Methods for establishing oral reference doses. In: Mertz W, Abernathy CO, & Olin SS eds. Risk assessment of essential elements. Washington, DC, ILSI Press, pp 51-61.

References

Dourson ML, Felter SP, & Robinson D (1996) Evolution of science-based uncertainty factors in noncancer risk assessment. Regul Toxicol Pharmacol, **24**: 108-120.

Fairweather-Tait SJ (1997) From absorption and excretion of minerals... to the importance of bioavailability and adaptation. Br J Nutr, **78**(suppl 2): S95-S100.

Fairweather-Tait SJ & Hurrell RF (1996) Bioavailability of mineral and trace elements. Nutr Res Rev, **54**: 295-324.

Feder JN, Gnirke A, Thomas W, Rsuchihashiu Z, Ruddy DA, Basava A, Dormishian F, Domingo R, jr, Ellis MC, Fullan A, Hinton LM, Jones NL, Kimmel BE, Kronmal GS, Lauer P, Lee VK, Loeb DB, Mapa FA, McClellan E, Meyer NC, Mintier GA, Moeller N, Moore T, Morikang E, Prass CE, Quintana L, Starnes SM, Schatzman RC, Brunke KJ, Drayna DT, Risch NJ, Bacon BR, & Wolff RK (1996) A novel MHC class I-like gene is mutated in patients with hereditary haemochromatosis. Nature Genetics, **13**: 399-408.

Fischer JG, Tackett RL, Howerth EW, & Johnson MA (1992) Copper and selenium deficiencies do not enhance the cardiotoxicity in rats due to chronic doxorubicin treatment. J Nutr, **122**: 2128-2137.

Forbes GB (1996) Body composition. In: Ziegler EE & Filer LJ eds. Present knowledge in nutrition. Washington, DC, ILSI Press, pp 7-12.

Frey H (1995) Iodine. In: Oskarsson A, ed. Risk evaluation of essential trace elements - essential versus toxic levels of intake. Copenhagen, Nordic Council of Ministers, pp 121-132.

Gaylor D, Ryan L, Krewski D, & Zhu Y (1998) Procedures for calculation of benchmark doses for health risk assessment. Regul Toxicol Pharmacol, **28**: 150-164.

Gunshin H, MacKenzie B, Berger UV, Gunshin Y, Romero MF, Nussberger S, Gollan JL, & Hediger MA (1997) Cloning and characterization of a mammalian proton-coupled metal-ion transporter. Nature, **388**: 482-488.

Heresi G, Castillo-Duran C, Munoz C, Arevalo M, & Schlesinger L (1985) Phagocytosis and immunoglobulin levels in hypocupremic infants. Nutr Res, **5**: 1327-1334.

Hetzel BS (1989) The story of iodine deficiency: an international challenge to nutrition. Oxford, Oxford University Press.

IAEA (1992) Human dietary intakes of trace elements: a global literature survey mainly for the period 1970-1991 I. Data list and sources of information. Vienna, International Atomic Energy Agency.

ILSI (1992) Similarities and differences between children and adults: implications for risk assessment. Guzelian PS, Henry CJ, & Olin S eds. Washington, DC, ILSI Press, pp 79-94.

ILSI (1994) Risk assessment of essential elements. Mertz W, Abernathy CO, & Olin SS, eds. Washington, DC, ILSI Press.

ILSI Proceeding of an ILSI Europe Workshop, Norwich, UK (1996) Assessment of the bioavailability of micronutrients. Eur J Clin Nutr, 1997, **51**(suppl 1): S1-S90.

IOM (Institute of Medicine) (2001) Dietary Reference Intakes: Vitamin A, Vitamin K, Arsenic, Boron, Chromium, Copper, Iodine, Iron, Manganese, Molybdenum, Nickel, Silicon, Vanadium, and Zinc. Washington DC, National Academy Press.

IPCS (1987) Environmental Health Criteria 70: Principles for the safety assessment of food additives and contaminants in food. Geneva, World Health Organization, International Programme on Chemical Safety.

IPCS (1990) Environmental Health Criteria 101: Methylmercury. Geneva, World Health Organization, International Programme on Chemical Safety.

IPCS (1992) Environmental Health Criteria 134: Cadmium. Geneva, World Health Organization, International Programme on Chemical Safety.

IPCS (1994) Environmental Health Criteria 170: Assessing human health risks of chemicals: derivation of guidance values for health-based exposure limits. Geneva, World Health Organization, International Programme on Chemical Safety.

IPCS (1998) Environmental Health Criteria 200: Copper. Geneva, World Health Organization, International Programme on Chemical Safety.

IPCS (1999) Environmental Health Criteria 210: Principles for the assessment of risks to human health from exposure to chemicals. Geneva, World health Organization, International Programme on Chemical Safety.

IPCS (2000) Environmental Health Criteria 214: Human exposure assessment. Geneva, World Health Organization, International Programme on Chemical Safety.

IPCS (2001) Environmental Health Criteria 221: Zinc. Geneva, World Health Organization, International Programme on Chemical Safety.

Jackson MJ, Jones DA, Edwards RH, Swainbank IG, & Coleman ML (1984) Zinc homeostasis in man. Studies using a new stable isotope dilution technique. Brit J Nutr, **51**: 199-208.

Johnson PE & Korynta ED (1992) Effects of copper, iron and ascorbic acid on manganese availability in the rat. Proc Soc Exp Biol Med, **200**: 470-480.

Kay RG, Tasman-Jones C, Pybus J, Whiting R, & Black HA (1976) A syndrome of acute zinc deficiency during total parenteral alimentation in man. Ann Surg, **183**: 331-340.

Keshan Disease Research Group of the Chinese Academy of medical science (1979) [Observations on the effect of sodium selenite in prevention of Keshan disease.] Chinese Medical Journal, **2**: 471-476 (in Chinese).

Klipstein-Grobusch K, Koster JF, Grobbee DE, Lindemans J, Boeing H, Hofman A, & Witteman JC (1999) Serum ferritin and risk of myocardial infarction in the elderly: the Rotterdam Study. Am J Clin Nutr, **69**: 1231-1236.

Kumpulainen J & Aro A (1995) Chromium. In: Oskarsson A ed. Risk evaluation of essential trace elements: essential versus toxic levels. Copenhagen, Nordic Council of Ministers, pp 133-143.

References

Kushner J (1985) Hypochromic anemias. In: Wyngaarden JB & Smith LH Jr. eds. Cecil textbook of medicine. Philadelphia, W.B.Saunders Co, pp 885-892.

Lin JX (1989) [Selenium treatment to prevent Kashin-Beck disease.] Chinese J Epidemiology, **4**: 27-30 (in Chinese).

Liuzzi JP, Blanchard RK, & Cousins RJ (2001) Differential regulation of zinc transporter 1, 2, and 4 mRNA expression by dietary zinc in rats. J Nutr, **131**: 46-52.

McKie AT, Marciani P, Rolfs A, Brennan K, Wehr K, Barrow D, Miret S, Bomford A, Peters TJ, Farzaneh F, Hediger MA, Hentze MW, & Simpson RJ (2000) A novel duodenal iron-regulated transporter, IREG1, implicated in the basolateral transfer of iron to the circulation. Molecular Cell, **5**: 299-309.

Mertz W ed (1987) Trace elements in human and animal nutrition, 5th edition, Vols 1 & 2. San Diego, Academic Press.

Mertz W (1993) Essential trace metals: new definitions based on new paradigms. Nutr Rev, **51**: 287-295.

Mertz W, Abernathy CO, & Olin SS eds. (1994) Risk assessment of essential elements. Washington, DC, ILSI Press.

Mertz W (1998) A perspective on mineral standards. J Nutr, **128**: 375S-378S.

Mills CF (1985) Dietary interactions involving trace elements. Ann Rev Nutr, **5**: 173-193.

Moore MR, McCall KEL, Rimington C, & Goldberg A (1997) Disorders of porphyrin metabolism. New York, Plenum Press.

Müller T, Müller W, & Feichtinger H (1998) Idiopathic copper toxicosis. Am J Clin Nutr, **67**(5 suppl): 1082S-1086S.

National Iodine Deficiency Disorder (IDD) Surveillance Group (2000) [An analysis of surveillance data on IDD in 1999 in China.] Chinese J Epidemiology, **19**: 269-271 (in Chinese).

Niederau C, Fische R, & Sonnenberg A (1985) Survival and causes of death in cirrhotic and noncirrhotic patients with primary hemochromatosis. N Engl J Med, **313**: 1256-1262.

Nordberg GF & Skerfving S eds (1993) Biological monitoring, carcinogenicity and risk assessment for essential trace elements. Scand J Work Environ Health, **19**(suppl 1):1-140.

Nordberg M & Nordberg GF (2000) Toxicological aspects of metallothionein. Cellular and molecular biology, **46**: 451-463.

NRC (1989) Recommended dietary allowances. Washington, DC, National Academy Press.

O'Donnell T (1997) Zinc and health-conclusions of the Health Working Group. In: Langley A & Mangas S, eds. Report of an International Meeting, September 1996. Adelaide, South Australian Health Commission, pp 68-75.

Olin SS (1998) Between a rock and a hardplace: methods for setting dietary allowances and exposure limits for essential minerals. J Nutr, **128**: 364S-367S.

Oskarsson A ed. (1995) Risk evaluation of essential trace elements: essential versus toxic levels of intake. Report of a Nordic Project. Copenhagen, Nordic Council of Ministers, 185 pp.

Oskarsson A & Sandstrom B (1995) A Nordic project - risk evaluation of essential elements: essential versus toxic levels of intake. Analyst, **120**: 911-912.

Pena MM, Lee J, & Thiele DJ (1999) A delicate balance: homeostatic control of copper uptake and distribution. J Nutr, **129**: 1251-1260.

Picciano MF (1996) Pregnancy and lactation. In: Present knowledge in nutrition, 7th edition. Washington, DC, ILSI Press, pp 384-395.

Pieters MN, Kramer HJ, & Slob W (1998) Evaluation of the uncertainty factor for subchronic-to-chronic extrapolation: statistical analysis of toxicity data. Regul Toxicol Pharmacol, **27**: 108-111.

Prasad AS (1998) Zinc deficiency in humans: a neglected problem. J Am Coll Nutr, **17**: 542-543.

Robinson MF (1989) Selenium in human nutrition in New Zealand. Nutr Rev, **47**: 99-107.

Sandstead H (1993) Zinc requirements, the recommended dietary allowance and the reference dose. Scand J Work Environ Health, **19**: 128-131.

Sandstead HH (1995) Requirements and toxicity of essential trace elements, illustrated by zinc and copper. Am J Clin Nutr, **61**(suppl): 621S-624S.

Sandström B (1998) Toxicity considerations when revising the Nordic nutrition recommendations. J Nutr, **128**: 372S-374S.

SCF (2000) Guidelines of the Scientific Committee on Food for the development of tolerable upper intake levels for vitamins and minerals. European Commission, Health and Consumer Protection Directorate-General. Report SCF/CS/NUT/UPPLEV/11 Final. Brussels, 11 pp.

Scholl TO & Hediger ML (1994) Anemia and iron-deficiency anemia: compilation of data on pregnancy outcomes. Am J Clin Nutr, 59(suppl. 2): 492S-500S.

Scholl TO, Salmon RW, & Miller LK (1986) Smoking and adolescent pregnancy outcome. J Adolesc Health Care, **7**: 390-394.

Schümann K, Classen HG, Hages M, Prinz-langenohl R, Pietrzik K, & Biesalski HK (1997) Bioavailability of oral vitamins, minerals, and trace elements. Arzneim-Forsch/Drug Res, **47**: 369-380.

Shaw JCL (1992) Copper deficiency in term and preterm infants. In: Fomon SJ & Zlotkin S eds. Nutritional anemias. New York, Raven Press, Nestlé Workshop Series, **30**: 105-119.

References

Solomons NW, Rosenberg IH, & Sandstead HH (1976) Zinc nutrition in coeliac sprue. Am J Clin Nutr, **29**: 371-375.

Stanbury JB (1996) Iodine deficiency and the iodine deficiency disorders. In: Ziegler EE & Filer LJ eds. Present knowledge in nutrition. Washington, DC, ILSI Press, pp 378-383.

Sternlieb I (1980) Copper and liver. Gastroenterol, **78**: 1615-1628.

Stevens R (1996) Excess iron and risk of cancer. In: Allberg L & Asp N-G eds. Iron nutrition in health and disease. London, John Libby and Co., pp 278-284.

Suzuki KT, Tamagawa H, Takahashi K, & Shimojo N (1990) Pregnancy-induced mobilization of copper and zinc bound to renal metallothionein in cadmium loaded rats. Toxicol, **60**: 199-210.

Telisman S (1995) Interactions for essential and/or toxic metals and metalloids regarding interindividual differences in susceptibility to various toxicants and chronic diseases in man. Arh Hig Rada Toksilkol, **46**: 459-476.

Tuomainen TP, Punnonen K, Nyyssonen K, & Salonen JT (1998) Association between body iron stores and the risk of acute myocardial infarction in men. Circulation, **97**: 1461-1466.

Turnlund JR, Durkin N, Costa F, & Margen S (1986) Stable isotope studies of zinc absorption and retention in young and elderly men. J Nutr, **116**: 1239-1247.

Turnlund JR, Keyes WR, Anderson HL, & Accord LL (1989) Copper absorption and retention in young men at three levels of dietary copper by use of the stable isotope ^{65}Cu. Am J Clin Nutr, **49**: 870-878.

Turnlund JR, Keyes WR, & Peiffer GL (1995) Molybdenum absorption, excretion, and retention studied with stable isotopes in young men at five intakes of dietary molybdenum. Am J Clin Nutr, **62**: 790-796.

Turnlund JR, Keyes WR, Peiffer GL, & Scott KC (1998) Copper absorption, excretion, and retention by young men consuming low dietary copper determined by using the stable isotope ^{65}Cu. Am J Clin Nutr, **67**: 1219-1225.

US EPA (1992) Guidelines for exposure assessment. Washington, DC, US Environmental Protection Agency, Office of Research and Development, Office of Health and Environmental Assessment (EPA/600/Z-92/001).

Vallee BL, Wacker WEC, Bartholomay AF, & Hoch FL (1957) Zinc metabolism in hepatic dysfunction, II. Correlation of metabolic patterns with biochemical findings. N Engl J Med, **257**: 1055-1065.

Walter TDE, Andraca I, Chadud P, & Perales CG (1989) Iron deficiency anaemia: adverse effects on infant psychomotor development. Pediatrics, **84**: 7-17.

Warkany J & Petering HG (1972) Congenital malformation of the central nervous system in rats produced by maternal zinc deficiency. Teratology, **5**: 319-334.

WHO (1996) Trace elements in human nutrition and human health. Geneva, World Health Organization.

WHO (2001) Biomarkers validity and validation. International programme on Chemical Safety and Environmental Health Criteria Vol. 222. Geneva, World Health Organization.

Yadrick MK, Kenney MA, & Winterfeldt EA (1989) Iron, copper and zinc status: response to supplementation with zinc or zinc and iron in adult females. Am J Clin Nutr, **49**: 145-150.

Yang GQ, Yin S, & Zhou R (1989a) Studies of safe maximal daily dietary Se-intake in a seleniferous area in China. 2. Relation between Se-intake and manifestations of clinical signs and certain biochemical alterations in blood and urine. J Trace Elem Electrolytes Health Dis, **3**: 123.

Yang GQ, Zhou R, & Yin S (1989b) Studies of a safe maximum daily dietary Se-intake in a seleniferous area in China. 1. Selenium intake and tissue selenium level of inhabitants. J Trace Electrolytes Health Dis, **1**: 77.

Yang YX & Chen XC (1993) [Impact of zinc intake on pregnant and lactating women and newborn and infant development.] Acta Nutrimenta Sinica, **15**: 415-419 (in Chinese).

Yip R & Dallman PR (1996) Iron. In: Ziegler EE & Filer LJ eds. Present knowledge in nutrition. Washington, DC, ILSI Press, pp 277-292.

Younes M, Meek ME, Hertel RF, Gibb H, & Schaum J (1998) Risk assessment and management. In: Herzstein JA, Bunn WB, Fleming LE, Harrington JM, Jeyaratnam J, & Gardner IR eds. International Occupational and Environmental Medicine. St. Louis, Mosby, pp 62-74.

Zhang KL (1998) [Keshan Disease.] In: Geng GY ed. Epidemiology vol 3, 2nd edition. People's Publishing House, Beijing, pp 378-397 (in Chinese).

Ziegler EE & Filer LJ Jr, eds. (1996) Present knowledge in nutrition, 7th edition. Washington, DC, ILSI Press, 684 pp.

Zhu Y & Haas J (1997) Iron depletion without anemia and physical performance in young women. Am J Clin Nutr, **66**: 334-341.

RESUME

La méthode basée sur l'évaluation du risque qui est décrite dans cette monographie ne s'applique qu'aux oligo-éléments essentiels à la santé humaine, à l'exclusion des éléments non essentiels. La monographie a pour objet d'exposer les méthodes dans le cadre desquelles il est possible d'analyser la démarcation entre un apport insuffisant et un apport excessif d'oligo-éléments essentiels par voie orale. L'application des principes décrits dans la monographie nécessite une évaluation scientifique pluridisciplinaire, sur la base des données relatives aux apports nutritifs, insuffisants ou excessifs.

La monographie est centrée sur la notion de fourchette acceptable d'apport par voie orale (ou *acceptable range of oral intake, AROI*). L'AROI a été conçue pour limiter les apports insuffisants ou excessifs d'oligo-éléments dans les populations en bonne santé et sa valeur est fixée en fonction du sexe et de la tranche d'âge des sujets ou selon des critères physiologiques comme la grossesse ou l'allaitement. Pour faciliter les comparaisons, les AROI sont discutées par rapport à d'autres méthodes d'évaluation du risque.

L'absorption, l'excrétion et la rétention tissulaires sont sous la dépendance de mécanismes homéostatiques qui permettent l'adaptation de l'organisme à la variation des apports en nutriments. Ces mécanismes assurent l'apport systémique optimal nécessaire à l'accomplissement des fonctions essentielles et il faut en tenir compte lors de l'établissement d'une AROI. L'influence d'autres facteurs, comme la forme chimique, les caractéristiques diététiques et les interactions des oligo-éléments essentiels est également déterminante pour l'établissement des AROI correspondantes.

Lorsque l'apport en oligo-éléments se situe en dehors de la fourchette représentée par l'AROI, l'homéostase ne peut plus jouer son rôle régulateur et la probabilité d'effets indésirables augmente. Le modèle homéostatique a été utilisé pour établir cette fourchette et il est illustré par des exemples et des courbes théoriques.

La première étape consiste dans le choix de la base de données relative à l'oligo-élément essentiel étudié. On procède ensuite à l'identification du danger en fonction des éléments de preuve dont on dispose, en choisissant les points d'aboutissement physiologiques pertinents d'un apport insuffisant ou au contraire excessif d'oligo-éléments essentiels. Après avoir calculé la probabilité du risque et déterminé la gravité des divers effets, on choisit les effets jugés déterminants, puis on établit l'AROI en établissant un équilibre entre les points d'aboutissement d'importance sanitaire comparable. C'est à ce stade qu'il est procédé à l'évaluation de l'exposition. Enfin, on passe à la caractérisation du risque en indiquant les points forts et les faiblesses des bases de données utilisées, compte tenu de l'AROI et de l'exposition.

RESUMEN

El método de evaluación de riesgos descrito en esta monografía se aplica sólo a los oligoelementos esenciales (OE) que contribuyen a la salud humana y no a elementos no esenciales. La monografía tiene por objeto facilitar métodos que ofrezcan un marco para determinar los límites entre ingestas orales deficientes y excesivas de OE. La aplicación de los principios descritos en esta monografía comprende una evaluación científica multidisciplinaria utilizando datos sobre la ingesta necesaria de nutrientes, la deficiencia de éstos y la exposición excesiva a los mismos.

Esta monografía concentra la atención en el concepto de margen aceptable de ingesta oral (MAIO). El MAIO está diseñado para limitar las ingestas deficientes y excesivas en la población sana y se establece para diferentes grupos de edad-sexo y diversos estados fisiológicos, como el embarazo y la lactancia. A fin de facilitar las comparaciones, el MAIO se examina en relación con otros métodos de evaluación de riesgos.

Los mecanismos homeostáticos comprenden la regulación de la absorción y la excreción, así como la retención tisular, que posibilitan la adaptación a diversas ingestas de nutrientes. Estos mecanismos prevén un suministro sistémico óptimo para el desempeño de las funciones esenciales y deben tenerse en cuenta a la hora de establecer un MAIO. La influencia de otros factores, como la forma química, las características del régimen alimentario y las interacciones entre OE, también es decisiva para determinar el MAIO de los OE.

Cuando las ingestas de OE están por encima o por debajo de los límites del MAIO, se rebasa la capacidad de los mecanismos homeostáticos y aumentan la probabilidad y la gravedad de los efectos adversos. El modelo homeostático se ha utilizado para establecer el MAIO y se ilustra con ejemplos y con una serie de curvas teóricas.

El proceso empieza con la selección de la base de datos para un OE específico. Luego se utiliza un método de ponderación de datos para la identificación de riesgos y se determinan los criterios de valoración pertinentes de las exposiciones deficiente y excesiva. Acto seguido se cuantifican la probabilidad de riesgo y la gravedad de diversos efectos y se seleccionan los efectos críticos. Luego se establece el MAIO sopesando los criterios de valoración de importancia comparable para la salud. En ese momento se procede a la evaluación de la exposición. Por último, se efectúa una caracterización de los riesgos determinando los puntos fuertes y débiles de las bases de datos, integrando el MAIO y la evaluación de la exposición.

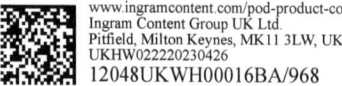
www.ingramcontent.com/pod-product-compliance
Ingram Content Group UK Ltd.
Pitfield, Milton Keynes, MK11 3LW, UK
UKHW022220230426
12048UKWH00016BA/968

9 789241 572286